Yoshiro Fujii

Dental treatment for whole body health

Yoshiro Fujii

Dental treatment for whole body health

LAP LAMBERT Academic Publishing

Imprint

Any brand names and product names mentioned in this book are subject to trademark, brand or patent protection and are trademarks or registered trademarks of their respective holders. The use of brand names, product names, common names, trade names, product descriptions etc. even without a particular marking in this work is in no way to be construed to mean that such names may be regarded as unrestricted in respect of trademark and brand protection legislation and could thus be used by anyone.

Cover image: www.ingimage.com

Publisher:
LAP LAMBERT Academic Publishing
is a trademark of
Dodo Books Indian Ocean Ltd. and OmniScriptum S.R.L publishing group

120 High Road, East Finchley, London, N2 9ED, United Kingdom
Str. Armeneasca 28/1, office 1, Chisinau MD-2012, Republic of Moldova, Europe
Managing Directors: Ieva Konstantinova, Victoria Ursu
info@omniscriptum.com

Printed at: see last page
ISBN: 978-3-659-74819-6

Dental treatment for whole body health

Yoshiro Fujii, DDS. Ph.D.

Introduction

I have been performing dental treatment which considers the health of the whole body. More specifically, I adjust biting situations to improve overall health. Conditions such as lumbago, stiffness of the shoulders and knee pain, which are sometimes difficult to cure, may be improved using this dental treatment. Moreover, a person who was bedridden may stand up suddenly and may begin to walk, after appropriate dentures are inserted. Such cases are clearly shown in the pictures and related movies. Please refer to Cases 2, 3, and 4. Teeth have a significant influence on the health of the whole body. It is not uncommon for illnesses or conditions which have no clear origin, to be related to dental problems. I began to suspect electromagnetic waves as another cause about ten years ago. In developed countries, societies are aging quickly. Since the elderly have reduced immunity and physical strength, intensive medical treatment is not used in most cases. Can't the elderly, who are bedridden and suffering from dementia, be saved any longer? The answer cannot be no. I think it is too early to give up. With suitable dental treatment, they may regain their health (Cases 7 and 8). Electromagnetic waves are more dangerous than most people think. The WHO (World Health Organization)/ International Agency for Research on Cancer (IARC) has classified radiofrequency electromagnetic fields as possible carcinogens to humans (Group 2B) based on an increased risk for glioma, a malignant type of brain cancer, associated with wireless phone use. The Supreme Court in Italy accepted a man's claim that long-term use of his cell phone at work was the cause of his brain tumor. The judgment relied on the research results of scholars in Sweden, who showed the relationship between cell phone use over many years and brain tumor development. If reducing medical expenses is necessary, nursing care expenses and the number of illnesses should be reduced.

And, the key to both is "dentistry."

Why I started my specific dental treatment.

I noticed the relationship between teeth and the whole body when I worked in a hospital for the elderly about 20 years ago. Before explaining the cases, I want to briefly explain the dental treatment which I have carried out. While working with the elderly, I observed many instances where the insertion of well-fitting dentures led to improvements in dementia and/or mobility. Those observations caused me to deeply believe that dental treatment is indispensable for maintaining and improving whole-body health. There are many hospitals in which patients' dentures are removed. An elderly person whose denture is removed may weaken rapidly, and may become bedridden. Removing a denture may cause dementia to worsen.   Although the purpose of hospitals is to cure patients, conditions related to aging may actually worsen after a patient enters the hospital. Many people think that the main purpose of teeth is to chew food. However, this is not the case. The main purpose of teeth is to support the whole body. Therefore, when a false tooth is removed, a patient may not be able to walk and their body may weaken. Biting situation has a serious influence on the muscles and skeleton of the whole body. As proof, I found that people with contorted backbones have poor biting situations. The jaw bone tends to directly influence the backbone. Moreover, if the backbone contorts, the pelvis will be influenced. I have treated many elderly people. The tendency is for people with good biting situations to have a high QOL (quality of life) score or ADL (activities of daily living) score. On the other hand, there is also data that shows bedridden people have fewer remaining teeth. Therefore, we can maintain the body's ability to support it by inserting well-fitting dentures when teeth are lost. The fact that poor biting condition can lead to spinal contortion is becoming common knowledge. When biting situation is corrected, posture may even become upright. A Japanese proverb says "Bad posture is the origin of 10.000 illnesses." So, tooth trouble may actually be the root cause of 10.000 illnesses! Maintaining good posture is important for maintaining overall health. When the pelvis and spine are aligned properly, the spine will exhibit an S-shaped curve. Proper spinal curvature helps maintain balance within the body. It affects skeletal structure, nerves, internal secretions and immunity. Of course, dental

4

treatment cannot cure all symptoms and all illnesses. However, dental treatment can cure the illnesses caused by oral ailments. For example, intractable arthritic pain may have developed from metastasis of cancer. Therefore, first of all, it is important to receive a medical specialist's diagnosis before trying dental treatment. If the cause is not clear or the symptom is not improving in spite of having received medical treatment from a specialist, then a dental problem may be considered as a cause.

Features of my treatment

My dental treatment is almost the same as the dental treatment which other dentists are conducting. Although the procedures are the same, the purpose is a little different. I consider my patient's overall health when treating them. During my treatment, I diagnosis the patient's ailment using the Bi-Digital O-Ring Test or the SLR test. Then I use manipulation techniques to adjust the body joints, along with standard dental treatment, to treat the ailment. Let me explain these techniques in more detail. Along with the following explanations, you can see examples of each procedure on the attached DVD.

Three kinds of features of the treatment

① Using the Bi-Digital O-Ring Test

In order to find the right biting position, the most appropriate jaw position for the patient's health should be found. I use the O-ring test to do this. During the 1960's a new system of evaluation began to develop in Chiropractics. Dr George Goodheart DC found that evaluation of normal and abnormal body function could be accomplished using muscle power tests. Since the original discovery, the principle has broadened to include evaluation of the nervous, vascular, and lymphatic systems, nutrition, acupuncture, and cerebrospinal fluid function. This system is called "Applied Kinesiology". In the late 1970s Professor Yoshiaki Omura developed a new method of diagnosing and treating ailments based on Applied Kinesiology. He called his technique the O-ring test. The principal behind the O-ring test is that when we are depressed, our muscle power decreases. Similarly, muscle power will decrease when a point on the body, at which some problem is occurring, is stimulated. Conversely, when we feel mentally and/or physically healthy, our muscular power will increase. It is with the O-ring test that we can judge what is good or bad for the body by assessing the body's reaction. This is a very sensitive diagnostic method. Therefore, it can detect conditions that the patient is not even aware of. It is a very useful method for assessing whole-body conditions. When evaluating the oral area, the O-ring test is able to not only determine the correct jaw position, but also judge the quality of dental materials, as well as the form and color of the denture suited to the patient. When I make a denture or adjust biting situations, I find the ideal biting situation using this test.

References

1) OMURA YOSHIAKI, "Bi-digital O-ring test for imaging and diagnosis of internal organs of a patient", published 1993-02-23, issued 1993-02-23. US patent 5188107, http://academic.reed.edu/economics/parker/f11/354/pat/o-ring.pdf (last checked: 2/16 /2015)

2) http://bdort.org/ (last checked: 16 Feb 2015)

② Research using the SLR（Straight Leg Raising）test.

The SLR test is commonly used in orthopedics to diagnose the cause of lower-back, buttock and thigh pain resulting from herniated disks, sciatica, etc. During the test, the patient lays down on his/her back. Then, the person conducting the test raises the leg while ensuring the leg is straight. The test evaluates how far the leg can be raised before the patient feels pain and/or the person conducting the test feels tension.

Moreover, hip joint flexibility is also evaluated using knee abduction or adduction. The stiffer the joint, the worse the condition. The motion of the pelvic circumference joints (sacroiliac joints, hip joints, etc.) is closely related to the function of the jaw joint. I often carry out SLR tests to assess a patient's condition before or after treatment. When the biting situation is corrected, the whole skeletal structure including the pelvic circumference joints will move into proper alignment. As a result of this realignment, the degree by which the leg can be raised increases, and variations in flexibility between the left and right legs decreases (Figure1).

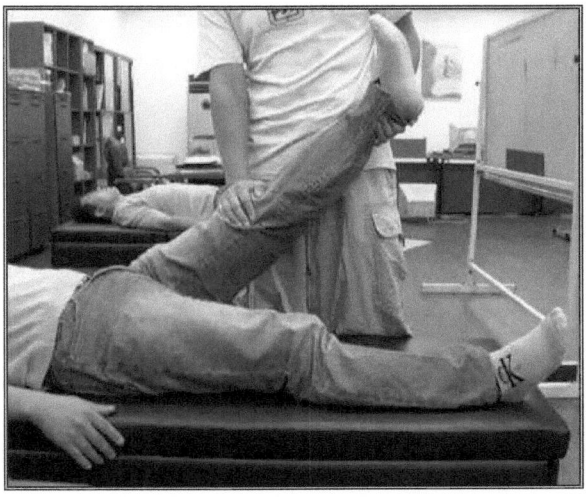

Figure 1: SLR test; Cited from (http://blog.daum.net/todj07/4563922)

③ Skeletal adjustment using the AKA (Arthrokinematic Approach Hakata method)

Biting situation is deeply related to overall skeletal alignment and therefore, has a great impact on the health of the whole body. Therefore, all dentists should have knowledge of the skeletal structure of the whole body. They should also perform their treatments with concern for the condition of the patient's whole body. When

7

diagnosing patients, I am always concerned with whole-body skeletal alignment. I ask my patients whether they have lumbago, stiffness of the shoulders, pain in the knees, or pain in the hip joints, etc. If required, I will adjust the skeletal alignment of the whole body with the AKA method. Since both the SLR test and the AKA method require the patient to lay down, a bed is needed. Therefore, dental offices should have beds. When I evaluate the patient's posture or adjust the body, it is the sacroiliac joint which I think is most important. The sacroiliac joint is a joint between the sacrum and ilium bones of the pelvis. Although it is fixed in place by many ligaments and does not move perceptively, the sacroiliac joint does move; just like the bones of the skull. Poor motion of the sacroiliac joint is an indication of joint imbalance throughout the body. If an evaluation of this portion cannot be performed, then treatment of temporomandibular disorders, which cause pain and result in difficulty opening the mouth, also becomes difficult. Many of the patients with temporomandibular disorders will certainly have lumbago and stiffness of the shoulders. In many such cases, adjustment of the sacroiliac joint using AKA is needed for successful treatment. If skeletal adjustment with the AKA and the bite adjustment are performed simultaneously, quite a positive result can be expected.

Case 1

The patient's temporomandibular disorder and lumbago were cured by simple dental treatment.

Subject, Method, and Result

The subject is a woman in her 20s. She was a TV reporter. Her chief complaint was a chronic lumbago and difficulty opening the mouth because of a temporomandibular disorder. She sometimes noticed a click when opening the mouth. I could not even place two fingers in her mouth when it was fully open (Figure 2). Moreover, when she tried to bend her back, it was too painful to bend very far (Figure 3). When the SLR (Straight Leg Raising) test was done, the right leg went up to 90 degrees, but the left leg did not go up as far as the right leg (Figure 4). When her left leg was rotated outward and inward, she felt tightness in her back. It seemed that the flexibility of her left sacroiliac joint and her left hip joints were poor. The result of the Bi-Digital O-Ring Test showed a problem with the lower left first molar. I ground the outside of the tooth slightly (Figure 5). After that, I could place three fingers in her mouth (Figure 6). She said she was able to open her mouth without any discomfort (Figure 6). Both legs rose easily and there was no longer any difference between the left and right legs when the SLR test was done. Both legs rose up to 120 degrees (Figure 7).Even when she leant back, there was no pain in her back (Figure 8).

As a result, the temporomandibular disorder, her difficulty opening her mouth, and the lumbago improved immediately. Moreover, although she leaned to the left when standing before my treatment (Figure 9), after the treatment, her posture improved and her backbone became straighter (Figure 10).

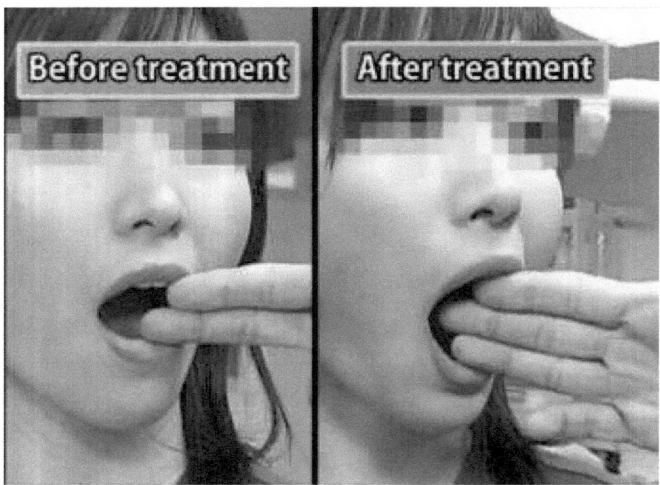

Figure 2   Figure 6

Figure 2: She could not open her mouth up to two fingers' width.

Figure 6: After grinding the buccal surface of her left lower first molar, she could open her mouth up to three fingers width.

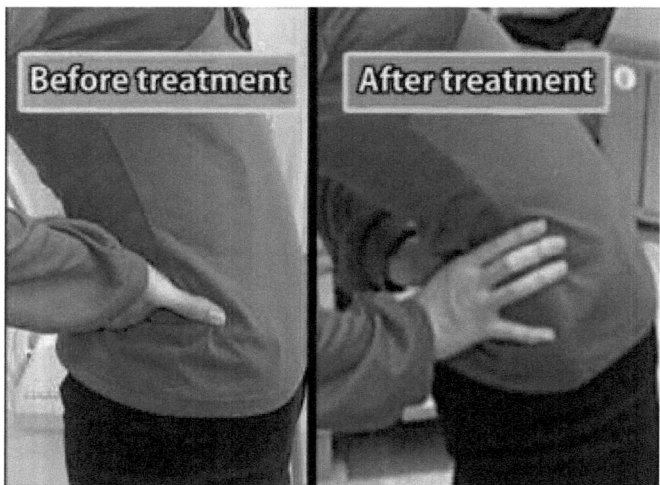

Figure 3   Figure 8

Figure 3: When she tried to bend back, it was too painful to bend very far.

Figure 8: Even when she bent back, there was no pain in her back after treatment.

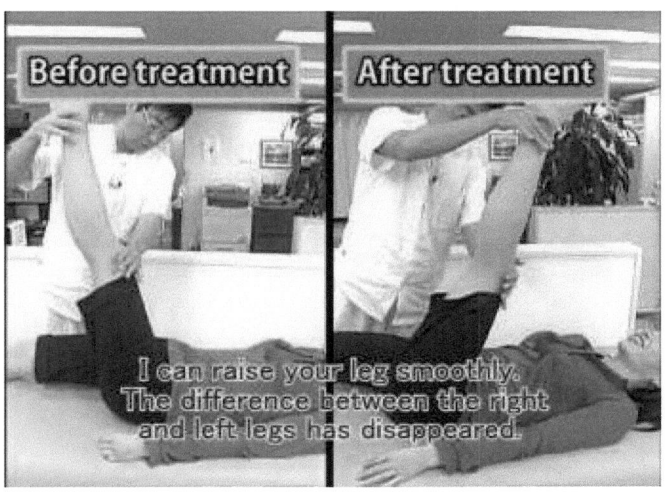

Figure 4   Figure 7

Figure 4: When the SLR (Straight Leg Raising) test was done, the right leg went up to 90 degrees, but the left leg went up to 80 degrees.

Figure 7: When the SLR test was done, there was no longer any difference between the left and right legs after treatment. Both legs rose up to 120 degrees

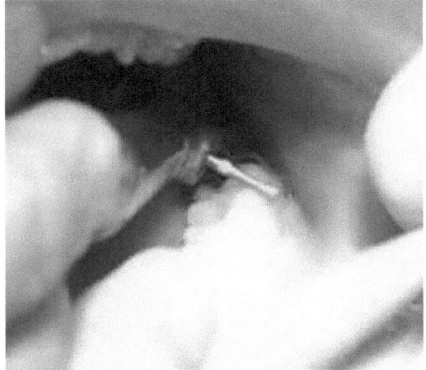

Figure 5: The buccal surface of her left lower first molar was ground.

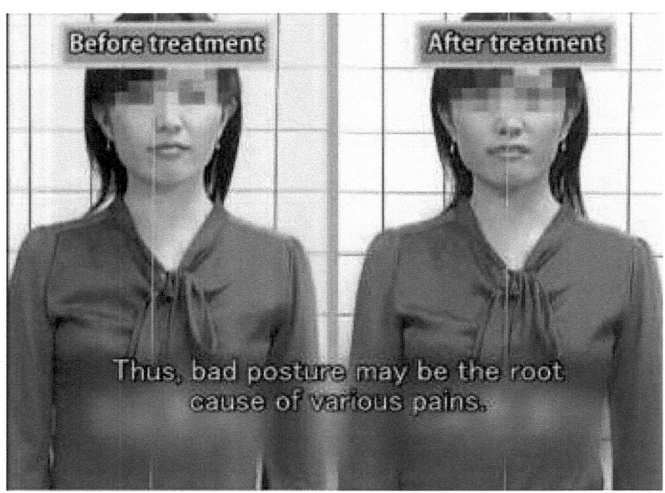

Figure 9   Figure 10

Figure 9: She leaned to the left when standing before my treatment.

Figure10:After the treatment, her posture improved and her backbone became straighter.

Discussion

Thus, chronic lumbago, which has continued for years, may be improved with simple dental treatment. Since the jaw supports the head, even small complications from biting condition may cause distortions of the spinal column, which can cause lumbago. If posture is poor, blood flow and lymphatic fluid flow will worsen and the nervous system and hormone levels will become unbalanced. Internal organs are also partially compressed by the misaligned spinal column which can reduce their ability to function.

Unnatural posture also causes chronic fatigue of the skeletal muscle of the whole body.

In the case of the female subject, her lumbago was improved, the symptoms of the temporomandibular disorder (i.e. her difficulty opening her mouth and the clicking of her jaw) were improved simultaneously.

This may be a typical case which illustrates that the mouth and the body should not be separated when we make a diagnosis. Therefore, don't separate a medical department and dentistry.

A simple tooth disorder may cause severe symptoms or lead to various illnesses.

However, modern medicine is only good at analyzing the part of the body where strong symptoms occur. There is a close relationship between dentistry and body posture.
Many patients suffer health problems due to the distortion of their posture, which is caused by dental disorders.

In order to watch the actual experiment described in this case, please visit the YouTube movie:
The temporomandibular joint disorder and lumbago were cured by simple dental treatment. https://www.youtube.com/watch?v=YiGd_AcUb_c

Case 2

The instep abnormality was improved by a single biting point adjust

Subject, Method, and Result

This treatment was performed at an international symposium taking place in Columbia University in New York. The subject was a woman in her 70's. She underwent her first operation 30 years ago due to a bone abnormality in her left instep. However, since the pain did not disappear, she tried various treatments, but her condition did not improve. Although she had had a second operation ten months before I treated her, her pain still did not disappear. She could still not put weight on her left leg. When I pushed her body from various directions, her body balance was very unstable (Figure 11).

13

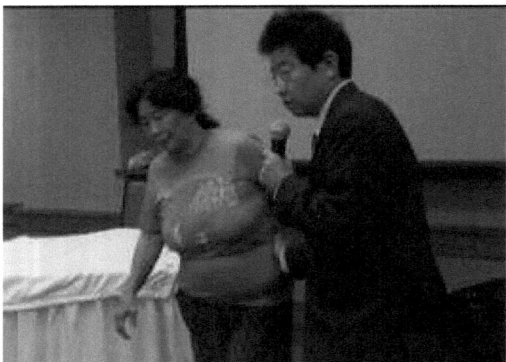

Figure 11: When she was pushed from the left side, her body balance was poor before treatment.

It seemed that her center of gravity was misaligned. When doing the SLR test, her left leg could barely be raised up to about 70 degrees, nor could it be raised up as high as her right leg (Figure 12).

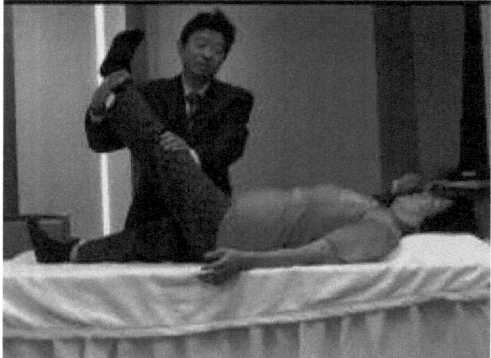

Figure 12: When doing the SLR test, her left leg could not be raised as high as her right leg

When raising her left leg, she also felt tension. When I examined her biting condition using the O-ring test, it turned out that the biting condition of her front tooth was abnormal i.e. when she bit the thin strip in her front teeth, her O-ring was opened easily (Figure 13). However, when she bit the strip in other tooth, her O-ring was not open (Figure 14).

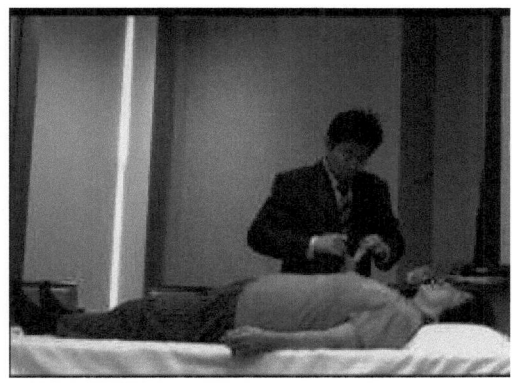

Figure 13: When she bit the thin strip in her front teeth, her O-ring was opened easily

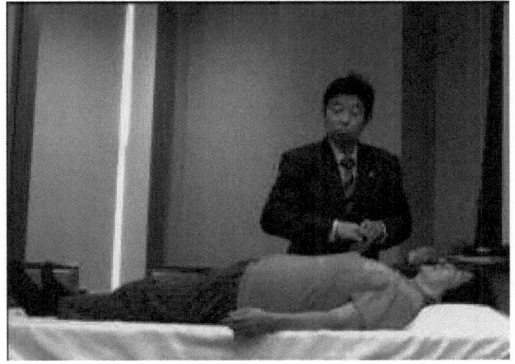

Figure 14: When she bit the strip in the other teeth, her O-ring was not open.

Therefore, the biter in her front tooth was adjusted until her O-ring was closed even when the strip was bitten in this position (Figure 15). Her SLR test results improved immediately after her biting condition was adjusted (Figure 16). Her center of gravity became aligned, so that when I pushed her, she was able to maintain her balance (Figure 17). The pain in her left leg was also reduced and it became easier for her to walk.

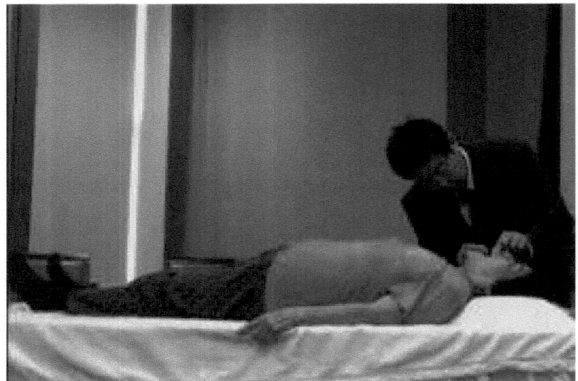

Figure 15: The bite in her front tooth biting was adjusted until her O-ring was closed even when the strip was bitten in this position

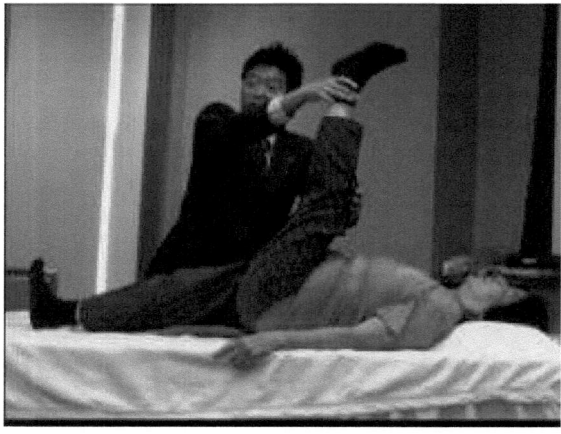

Figure 16: Her SLR test results improved immediately after her biting condition was adjusted

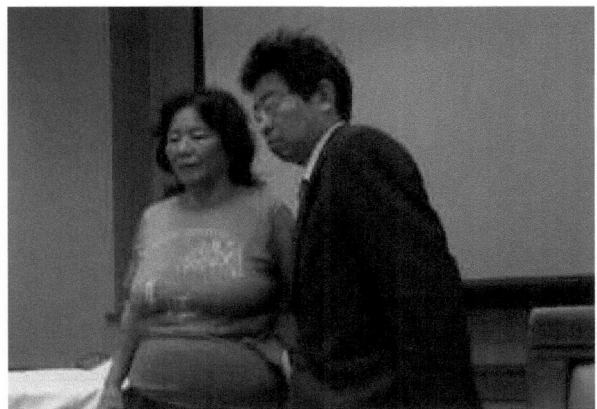

Figure 17: When she was pushed, she was able to maintain her balance after treatment.

Discussion

Misalignment of her center of gravity seems to have been the cause of her ailment. Her two operations had no effect on her condition because they did not align her center of gravity. Her center of gravity was improved by adjusting her biting situation. She became able to put weight on either leg equally. This might have caused her symptoms to improve. Modern Western medicine focuses on the specific areas where symptoms occur. This may prevent effective treatment because the root causes of ailments cannot always be identified in the specific area. The Bi-Digital O-Ring test may be useful to identify the root cause.

In order to watch the actual experiment described in this case, please visit the YouTube movie:

2012 NY Demonstration

https://www.youtube.com/watch?v=s35pViZvk-Q

Case 3

The symptoms of rheumatism were improved by simply placing one crown.

Subject, Method, and Result

The subject was a 67-year-old woman. She started to show the symptoms of rheumatoid arthritis in her late 30's. Therefore, she has suffered from the disease for about 30 years. Although slowly, the condition has gotten progressively worse. The joints of her fingers and toes were deformed (Figure 18). She was unable to stand up smoothly from a sitting position due to knee joint pain (Figure 19).

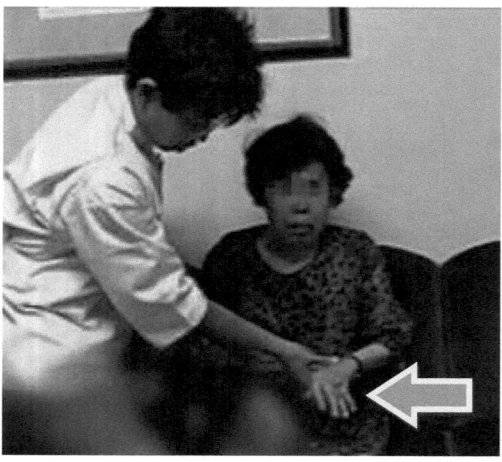

Figure 18: The joints of her fingers and toes were deformed (arrow).

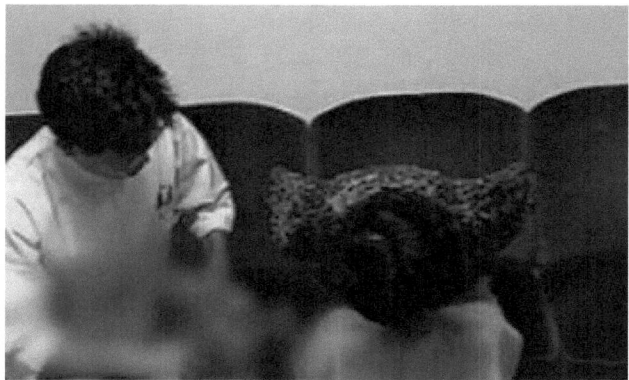

Figure 19: She was unable to stand up smoothly from a sitting position due to knee joint pain.

Although many of her teeth had been treated, almost all of her teeth remained and there was no impression that the biting condition was extremely bad. However, according to the O-Ring Test, the occlusal condition between the upper right first molar and the lower right first molar was insufficient. A gold alloy crown (it is mainly an alloy of gold and platinum) was set on the upper right first molar (Figure 20). The arthritic pain throughout her body decreased after that, and she no longer had difficulty rising out of a chair (Figure 21). Additionally, walking became easier. Thus, only a single tooth had a big influence on her entire body.

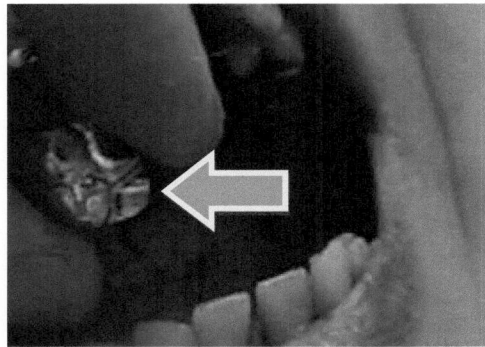

Figure 20: The crown which was set on her right upper first molar (arrow).

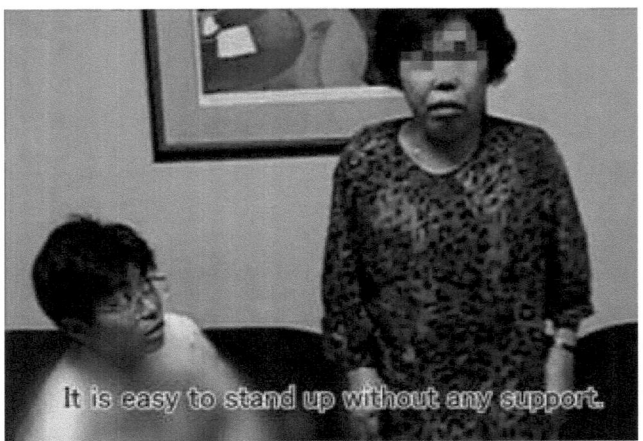

It is easy to stand up without any support.

Figure 21: She could stand up easily without any support after setting the crown.

Discussion

The purpose of teeth is not only to chew food. They may be organs, which are just as important as any other organ. The role of the mouth is not only to chew food. True health cannot be achieved unless we take this concept to heart. This book will introduce how dental treatment can be used to improve intractable diseases and symptoms, and to promote prompt recovery. Since dentistry looks at illnesses from a different viewpoint from standard medicine, a disease that may be recognized as intractable by medical doctors might be effectively treated by dentists.

However, with this case, there is a possibility, which was introduced in Case 16, which is that the peculiar wave motion of a substance can influence the body. When I began this treatment, I did not consider the effects of electromagnetic waves on the body, but based on my research, I am more concerned with it. It may have been possible for this subject to stand up by herself while simply holding the crown in her hand or having it somewhere near her body.

The pain throughout the subject's body was reduced immediately after placing the crown. This may seem impossible. If medical examinations are done just after the pain recedes, there will be no differences in the data obtained before and after the treatment. It is said that we understand what roles less than 10% of our genes perform. Conversely, there is a possibility, in such a case, that a certain change may have occurred, on the genetic level, immediately after dental treatment. Dental treatment might be effective on unknown diseases. Oral biting conditions influence the systems in our body. The cause of autoimmune disease, such as rheumatoid arthritis is unknown, so modern Western medicine has difficulty treating such diseases. The common medical treatment is to ease the symptoms using a steroid etc. The root cause of the disease is seldom treated. Dental treatment may be effective for treating rheumatoid arthritis; however, since the cause of the disease has not yet been clarified, it is difficult to explain how the treatment works. Many people still suffer from the symptoms of rheumatoid arthritis even after treatment using modern Western medical techniques. These people should consider dental treatment at least once.

In order to watch the actual experiment described in this case, please visit the YouTube movie:
The symptoms of rheumatism were improved by simply placing one crown.
https://www.youtube.com/watch?v=l399rOGS9Vo&feature=youtu.be

Case 4

A bedridden person was able to walk by herself for the first time in one year because of wearing proper fitting dentures.

Subject, Method, and Result

The subject was a 75 year-old woman experiencing paralysis due to a stroke. She experienced weakness and had trouble moving after the stroke. She was bedridden for

21

a year before treatment started. Although she could stand up, she could not walk without support, so she was placed in an institution for the handicapped. Although the left side of her body had light paralysis, her condition was not overly serious. There were no other particular symptoms besides her inability to walk. She did not have dentures although there were only several teeth in her upper and lower jaws (Figure 22, 23). So, she was fitted with upper and lower partial dentures (Figure 24), which allowed her to bite naturally (Figure 25). As soon as the dentures were set in her mouth, she started to walk without any help (Figure 26).

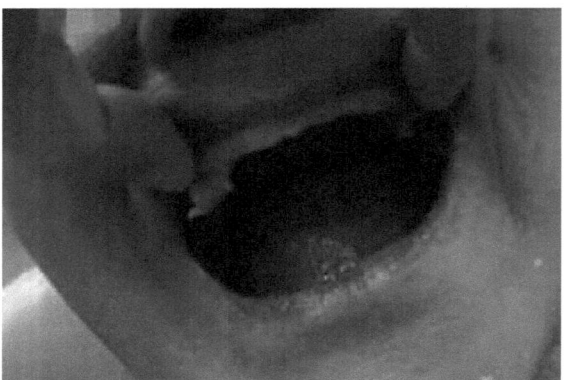

Figure 22: There were only a few teeth in her upper jaw.

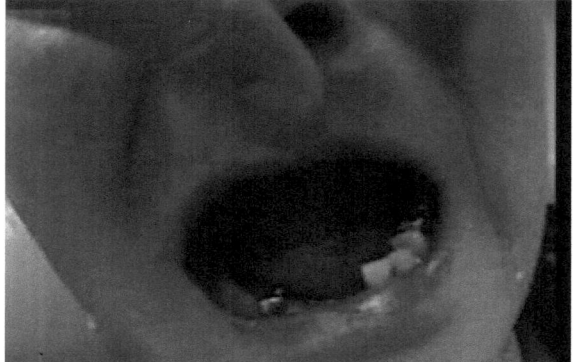

Figure 23: There were some teeth in her lower jaw.

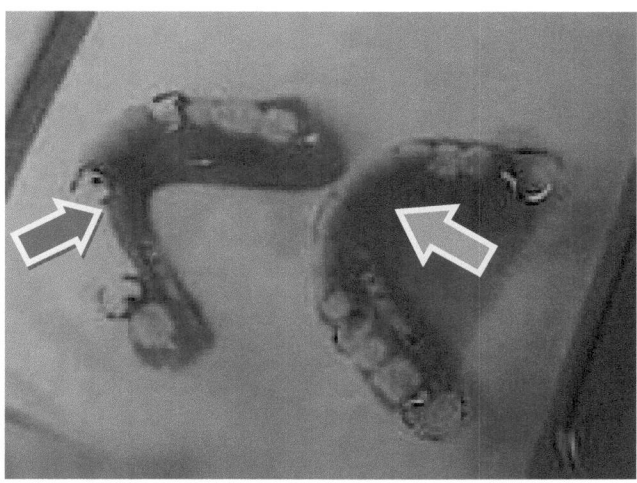

Figure 24: Her upper partial denture (right arrow) and lower partial denture (left arrow)

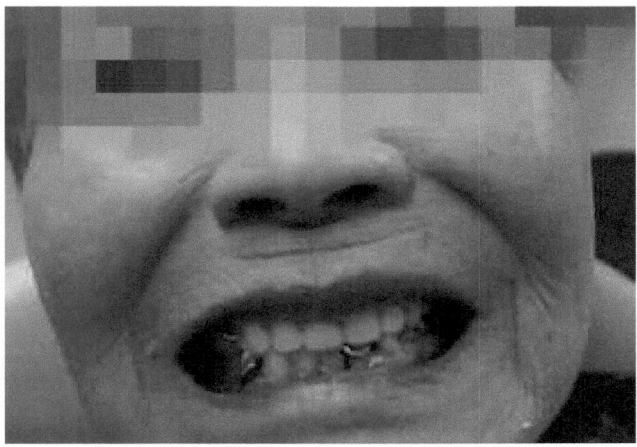

Figure 25: She became able to bite naturally after the dentures were placed in her mouth.

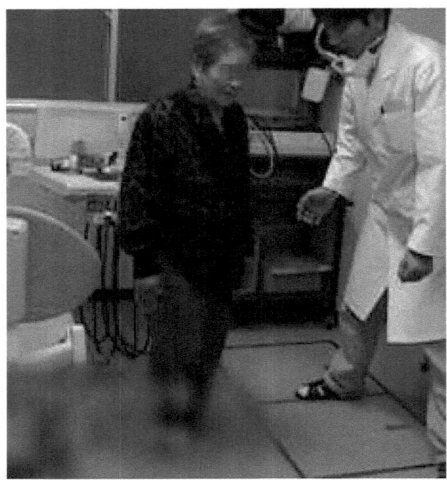

Figure 26: As soon as the dentures were set in her mouth, she started to walk without support.

She said "It is wonderful" and "I cannot believe it" because she walked by herself for the first time in one year. After finding that she was able to walk by herself she said "I'm surprised" with a happy expression on her face. Her dentures were adjusted once a week for one month. After one month, because she could easily walk by herself, the dental treatment was finished.

Discussion

In the case of this patient, I set the partial dentures painlessly. Moreover, no additional treatment (i.e. medication, rehabilitation, etc.) was used. The patient improved quickly. This shows that the body has a natural ability to recover without the aid of drugs or painful rehabilitation. There are important pressure points or reflexogenic zones in the sole.

These are stimulated automatically when walking. Such stimulation may be good for one's health. Conversely, bedridden patients do not experience this stimulation, which may cause rapid decline in their health. The denture treatment is very important in an aged society. As stated above, I worked at a geriatric hospital and was performing in-patient dental treatment.   The purpose of the dental treatment was not only to treat the teeth but also to rebuild systemic health. Bedridden elderly people stand up, and may begin to walk immediately following the insertion of well-fitting dentures. Although it may be hard to believe, such cases are not rare. It is not unusual for bedridden elderly people to be missing most, if not all, of their teeth. Despite this lack of teeth, few bedridden elderly people receive false teeth. When a false tooth is custom made and adjusted to fit a bedridden person well, how will its insertion influence the overall condition of the patient? Let's consider some specific examples.

In order to watch the actual experiment described in this case, please visit the YouTube movie:
A bedridden person was able to walk because of wearing dentures
https://www.youtube.com/watch?v=1vJiXlaR3M0

Case 5

The patient who had her denture removed in a hospital, saw her Quality of Life (QOL) decline.

Subject, Treatment, and Result

The subject was a 79-year-old woman. She could walk by herself with a cane when she came to the hospital. She was persuaded to remove her denture when she entered the hospital to have examinations. After that, her Quality of Life (QOL) declined rapidly. Although no particular abnormalities were discovered during the examinations, she became bedridden after her denture was removed. Her family wanted home care and moved her from the hospital. She recovered enough that she could eat soft food after some training. Although rehabilitation was also performed at home, she was not able to recover from her bedridden state. At this point, I was asked to visit her. When I began to carry out dental treatment in her home, the subject's condition was still getting worse and she was hardly conscious. She could not even open her eyes and she was completely bedridden. She could not change her body position by herself and she was unresponsive when her family spoke to her. She made chewing motions (oral dyskinesia) with her mouth, but did not speak. It seemed there was a possibility that she would die within 24 hours (Figure 27).

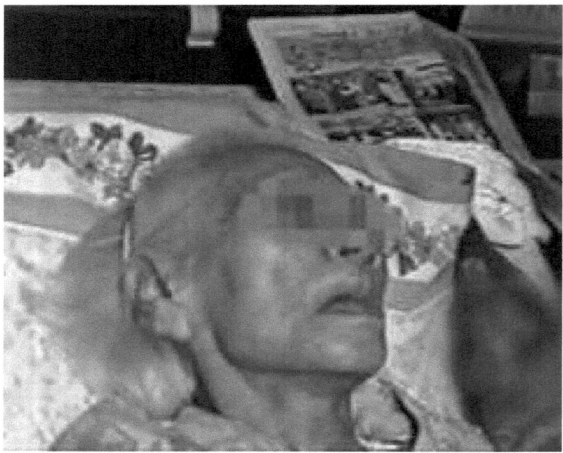

Figure 27: The subject was hardly conscious when the author visited her home for the first time. She could not even open her eyes and she was completely bedridden. It seemed there was a possibility that she would die within 24 hours.

The denture was still removed. It was difficult to replace the denture because her other teeth shifted while the denture was removed. So, I adjusted the denture and replaced it. Her eyes opened two weeks after the denture was replaced (Figure 28).

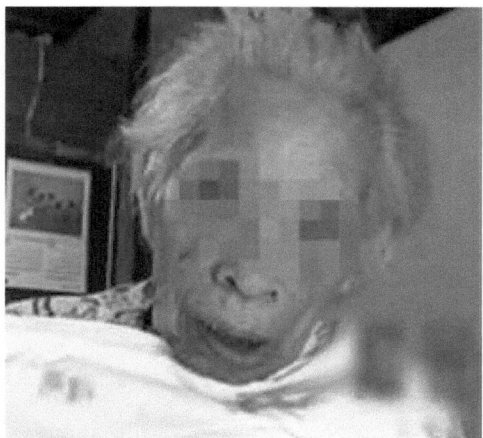

Figure 28: Her eyes opened two weeks after the denture was replaced.

She became able to eat soft food, and she regained some of her cognitive ability. Her QOL improved rapidly and her facial expressions began to show emotion (Figure 29). She recovered enough to perform rehabilitation on the side of the bed two months later.

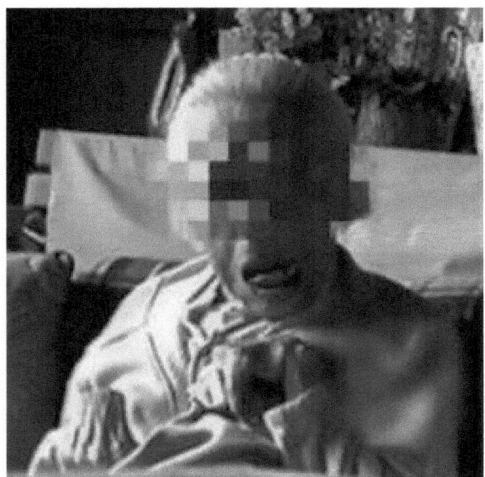

Figure 29: Her QOL improved rapidly and her facial expressions began to show emotion two months after replacing the denture.

Discussion

This case is not unique. Teeth or dentures are indispensable for the maintenance of normal life. The function of teeth is not only to facilitate eating, but also to support overall health. Tooth condition can influence bone alignment, which can lead to problems with related muscles. Furthermore, it affects nerve function, hormone balance and circulation of the blood, etc. Could it be that the problem is that the hospital suggested removing the denture? In this patient's case, she almost lost her life. Since a denture is an artificial organ, its removal can be damaging to the body, and therefore, inhumane. Removing dentures may sometimes be considered a murderous act. Dental treatment is sometimes the proper course of action to improve the overall health of someone like this. Additionally, the current case shows that a life-threatening crisis may be caused if the wrong dental treatment is administered. Due to the development of the Internet, many dental clinics now provide information on homepages. I think that an important criterion for the selection of a dental clinic should be whether or not the dentist is concerned with the whole body.

In order to watch the actual experiment described in this case, please visit the YouTube movie:
The patient who had her denture removed, saw her Quality of life decline.
https://www.youtube.com/watch?v=ox4NNtqM_UU&feature=youtu.be

Case 6

Spontaneous breathing can be restored soon after dental treatment in the intensive care unit (ICU).

Subject, Method, and Result

The subject was a 5 year-old boy. He was involved in a traffic accident. He was in a state of cardiopulmonary arrest for 30 minutes. Although his life was saved, spontaneous breathing did not occur because of a brain contusion. He was equipped with a respirator in the intensive care unit (ICU) of a university hospital (Figure 30).

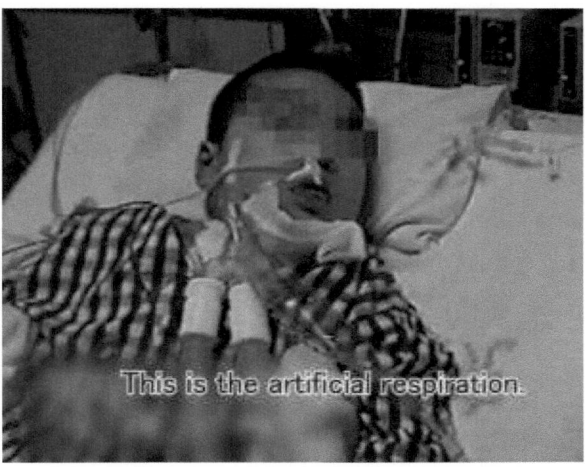

Figure 30: The subject was equipped with a respirator in the intensive care unit (ICU) of a university hospital.

He remained in this state for more than one month. The doctor in charge told his parents that there was almost no possibility of recovery, and that they should consider removing the respirator. However, if the respirator was removed, he would die within several minutes. When I visited him in the ICU, he was completely unconscious and he had almost no spontaneous breathing. The O-Ring Test was done using the fingers of his mother. His occlusion was adjusted and intraoral manipulation so that the morbid reaction of his head disappeared. In such a state, taking impressions and taking x-rays was impossible. About 5 minutes after finishing the dental treatment, his mother put her hand on his belly and said "It seems that he has begun to breathe on his own!" Then, his abdomen began to visibly move. Spontaneous breathing had restarted (Figure 31). The doctor in charge decided to remove the respirator four days later, and he was removed from the ICU (Figure 32).

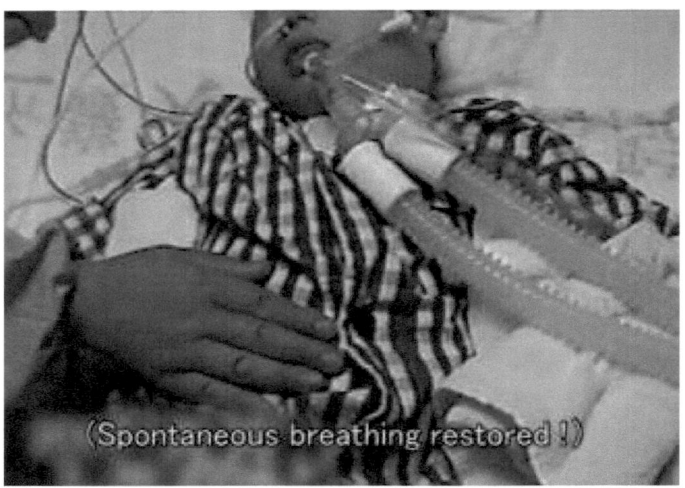

Figure 31: Spontaneous breathing had restarted about 5 minutes after dental treatment.

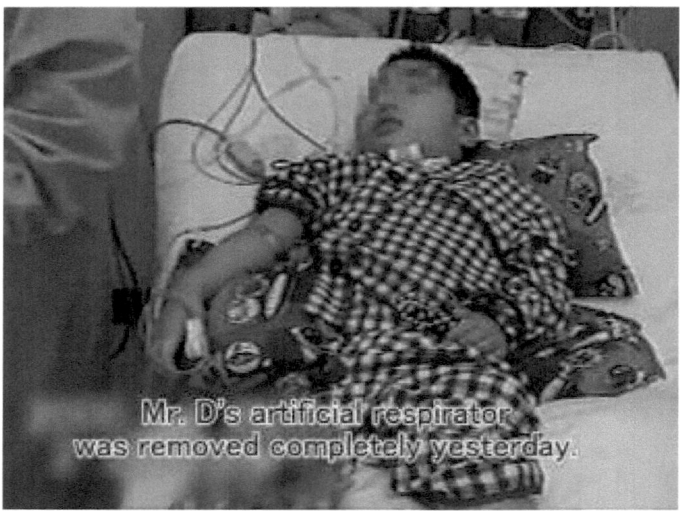

Figure 32: The doctor in charge decided to remove the respirator four days after the dental treatment.

Discussion

It is difficult to explain why his breathing recovered using modern scientific theories. I think his head had been deformed due to the pressure of the traffic accident. This deformation damaged the respiratory center of the brain. His skull deformation might have been reduced by the occlusal treatment and intraoral manipulation. Thus, the respiratory center recovered its function. Although dentists are not usually present during ER and ICU treatment, I think that dentists can play a large role in emergency medicine. I think that there is unnecessary loss of life in ERs and ICUs because there is not enough cooperation between dentistry and medicine.

There are many kinds of occlusal treatment. They are all based on different theories of treatment. If it is a mild case, I think that each treatment can be effective, but if it becomes a serious case, results will vary. Case 5 and Case 6, which will be introduced next, are life-threatening cases. When the patient is not conscious, X-ray diagnosis and verbal consultation with the patient are impossible. Taking dental impressions is also impossible. Since the patient in Case 6 was treated in an ICU, advanced dental care apparatus could not be brought in. The inability to administer advanced dental treatment in the ICU was a great disadvantage in this situation. If dentists using advanced dental care technology take part in the medical treatments in ERs or ICUs, I think that more people can be saved. Case 6 is one such case.
I think that it is necessary to train many dentists to do the dental treatments that were used in Cases 5 and 6.

In order to watch the actual experiment described in this case, please visit the YouTube movie:
Spontaneous breathing can be restored soon after dental treatment in ICU
https://www.youtube.com/watch?v=fdjC-i40JWc&feature=youtu.be

Case 7

Serious dementia may be cured by wearing a complete denture, Part 1.

Subject, Method, and Result

The subject was a woman in her 70's. She did not even know her name, nor where she was. When she came into the dental treatment room of the hospital, she began to wander around (Figure 33).

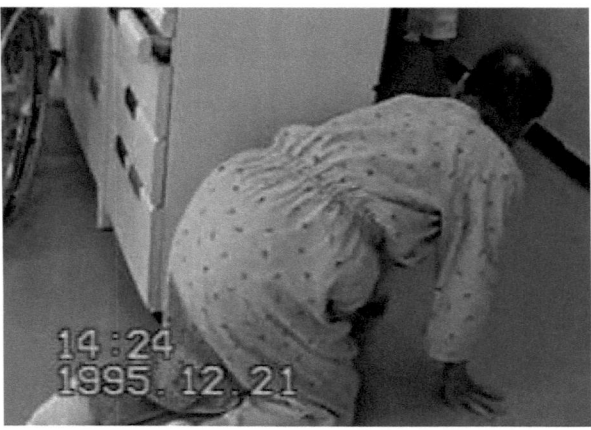

Figure 33: When she came into the dental treatment room of the hospital, she began to wander around

Although many upper teeth remained, she did not have any lower teeth. She was always moving her mouth (oral dyskinesia). Then, I made a lower full denture and placed it in her mouth (Figure 34).

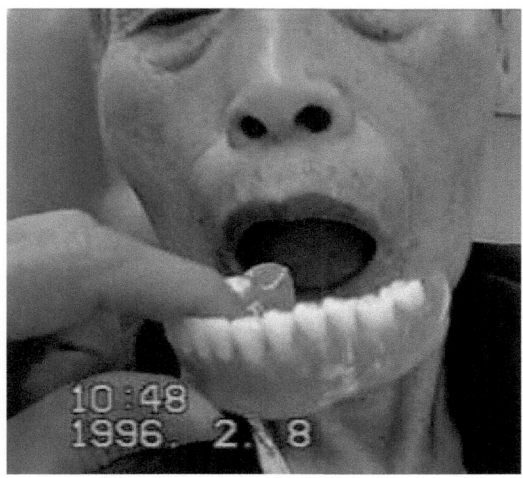

Figure 34: A lower full denture was placed in her mouth.

When I placed the full denture in her mouth, her oral movement stopped and her face brightened. Two weeks later, she had become more aware of her surroundings and was able to respond to the greeting "hello" (Figure 35).

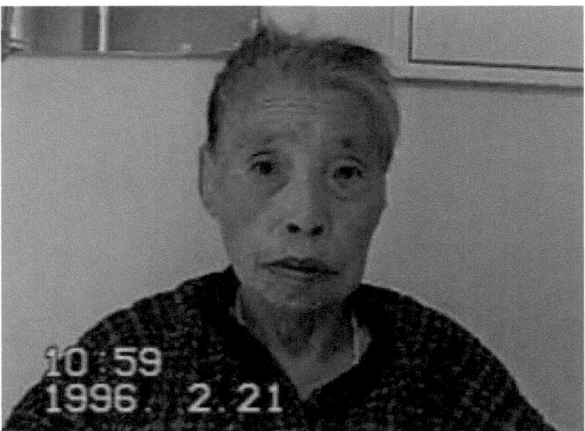

Figure 35: Two weeks after setting a lower full denture, she had become more aware of her surroundings and was able to respond to the greeting "hello".

However, when the denture was removed, her mouth movement started again, and her awareness dimmed rapidly. Five weeks later, she became able to have conversations naturally and she was also able to read the clock. Her words "I can now read a clock. Thank you" remain in my heart.

Discussion

I have treated many dementia patients with dentures. If it is light dementia, the condition may disappear within twenty-four hours of the insertion of the dentures. Although there is also medication for dementia, it is said that it only delays the progression of the ailment. However, dental treatment has been shown not only to delay progression, but also to reverse the progression of dementia in some cases. I think that this case illustrates how one's oral condition can have a direct influence on brain function.

In order to watch the actual experiment described in this case, please visit the YouTube movie:
Dental treatment for dementia Part 1
https://www.youtube.com/watch?v=2mVTzPBh8mY

Case 8

Serious dementia may be cured by wearing a complete denture, Part 2.

Subject, Method, and Result

The subject was a woman in her 70's. She always had her mouth open (Figure 36). Her dementia had progressed considerably.

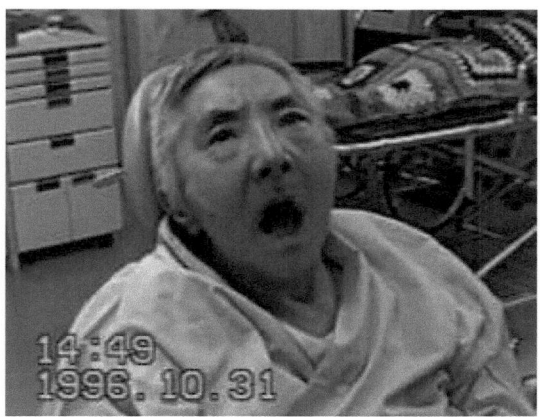

Figure 36: She always had her mouth open. She seemed to have serious dementia.

Although she had no teeth in her mouth, she didn't have any dentures. Many of those who cannot walk by themselves or are bedridden don't have a denture although they have many missing teeth. It is likely that there are also many people who need not have been hospitalized in a geriatric hospital, if suitable false teeth had been inserted in their mouths. I decided to make full dentures and place them in her upper and lower jaws. At first, I placed a full denture in her upper jaw. After placing the full denture in her upper jaw, she started to say "ahaaa…" It is not so rare for a patient's condition to change when even an upper full denture is placed in the mouth. The mechanism has not been clarified yet, but probably due to the deformation of the skull. Three weeks after putting in the upper full denture, the lower full denture was put in. The day on which the lower full denture was put in, was the last examination day of the year. Two weeks after placing the lower full denture, she seemed very steady and had become able to make a New Year's greeting and carry on daily conversation (Figure 37).

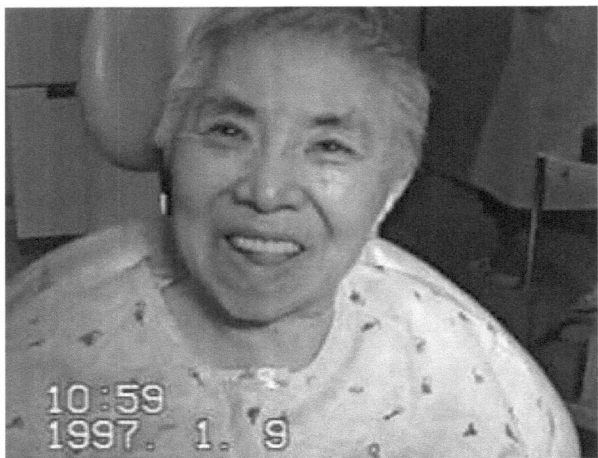

Figure 37: She seemed very steady and she could carry on daily conversation.

Although only two weeks had passed since the lower full denture was placed, she had a more normal facial expression which could not have been imagined when the serious dementia was causing her to open her mouth all the time.

Discussion

'Penfield's brain map' (refer to figure 38) shows which area of the cerebral sensory cortex are related to which parts of the body. This means that when a body part is stimulated, a certain part of the cerebral sensory cortex will be activated. In the figure, the picture of the body parts illustrates which parts of the cerebral sensory cortex they are linked to. As can be seen in the figure, the mouth and fingers activate large portions of the cerebral sensory cortex. 'Penfield's brain map' can help to explain the causes of Cases 7 and 8. Since the mouth has a great influence on the brain, treating the mouth can improve the mental state as well (Figure 38).

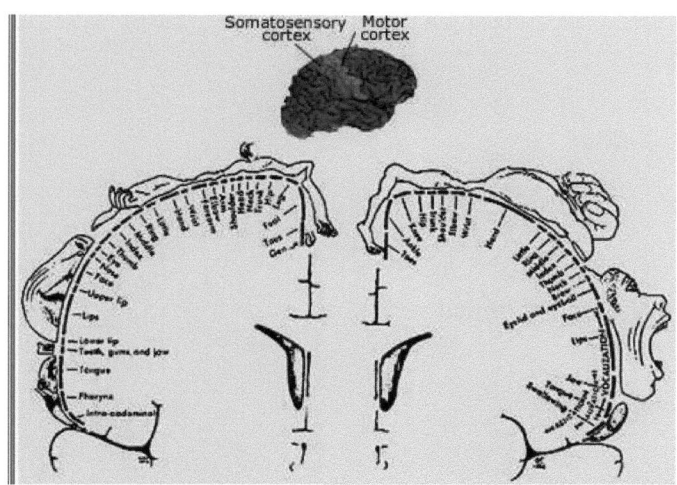

Figure 38: Mapping the Homunculus.

Citied by:

http://www.yproductions.com/writing/archives/mapping_the_urban_homunculus.html

There is no concrete explanation as to why dementia improves when dentures are inserted, but this gives us some clues. What cannot be overlooked in these two cases is that despite missing teeth, neither patient used dentures. I suggest that their dementia could have been prevented by the placement of suitable dentures. While dementia is becoming a more and more important issue as the population ages, dental treatment is also more important, so we may be able to reduce the number of dementia sufferers. You may have also heard that biting is a good stimulus for the brain. If you would like to prevent dementia, you should maintain your ability to bite. It is important to maintain your teeth through adequate dental treatment from a young age. The challenge of serious dementia dental treatment is sometimes effective on dementia as well as on the bedridden. It is said that it is difficult to recover from dementia once it sets in. Furthermore, it is judged that recovery is impossible in many cases of serious dementia. However, there is hope, dental treatment is sometimes effective in treating such serious dementia.

In order to watch the actual experiment described in this case, please visit the YouTube movie:

Dental treatment for dementia Part 2

https://www.youtube.com/watch?v=WfTnjYc-EzE

Case 9

Temporomandibular disorder due to malocclusions.

Subject, Method, and Result

The subject was a 24-year-old woman who had difficulty opening her mouth for several days before seeking treatment. She was only able to open her mouth the width of two fingers (Figure 39).

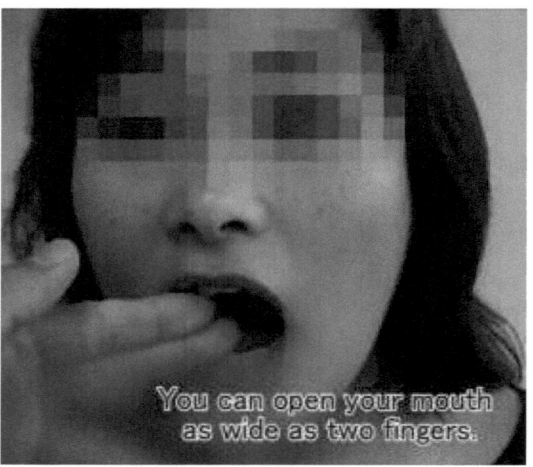

Figure 39: She was only able to open her mouth the width of two fingers

She experienced pain in the jaw, the head, and the shoulders. She said that her neck and shoulders felt hot. The pain and discomfort made it difficult for her to perform as usual. I diagnosed her with temporomandibular disorder (TMD) after examining her. I investigated the cause of her TMD using the O-ring test. As a result, I adjusted two of her teeth slightly i.e. the occlusal surface of the lower right second premolar and buccal surface and upper left second molar (Figure 40).

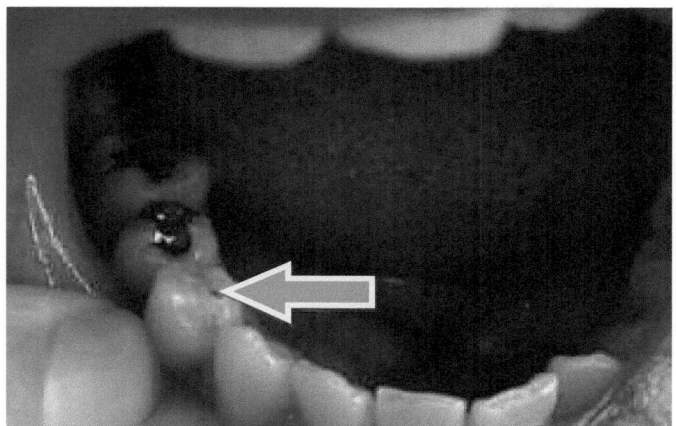

Figure 40: The occlusal surface of the lower right second premolar (arrow) and buccal surface and upper left second molar were adjusted

After the treatment, she was instantly able to open her mouth up to three fingers' width entirely (Figure 41). One finger's width is about 15 mm, so she could open her mouth about 45 mm. All of the pain in her head and shoulders disappeared simultaneously. Several days later, it had not recurred. She said she felt good. She was very satisfied.

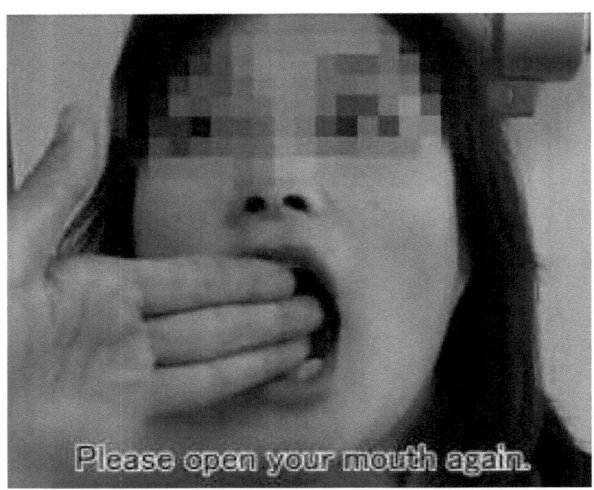

Figure 41: After the treatment, she was instantly able to open her mouth up to three fingers' width entirely.

Discussion

There is a close relationship between the temporomandibular joints and the other joints throughout the body. Have you heard of temporomandibular disorder (TMD)? The main symptoms of this illness are difficulty opening the mouth, as well as pain and clicking sounds when moving the jaw. Headaches, stiffness of the shoulders, neck pain, back pain, lumbago, etc. are known to be accompanying conditions. Although temporomandibular disorder is a functional disorder of the jaw joint, the function of jaw joints and other joints throughout the body are closely connected.

In order to watch the actual experiment described in this case, please visit the YouTube movie:

Temporomandibular disorder due to malocclusions.

https://www.youtube.com/watch?v=A8xOPJooTso

Case 10

Temporomandibular disorder caused by joint abnormalities in the lower body.

Difficulty opening the mouth was improved by adjustment of the joints of the back and foot.

Subject, Method, and Result

The subject was a woman in her twenties. She had a typical temporomandibular disorder. She had difficulties opening her mouth and had pain when she attempted to open her mouth. She could open her mouth only as wide as one and half fingers' width (Figure 42). Her jaw also made a clicking sound. She had a small jaw. She visited my dental clinic with a dark expression. When SLR (Straight Leg Raising) test was done, the patient felt pain and discomfort in her left leg (Figure 43).

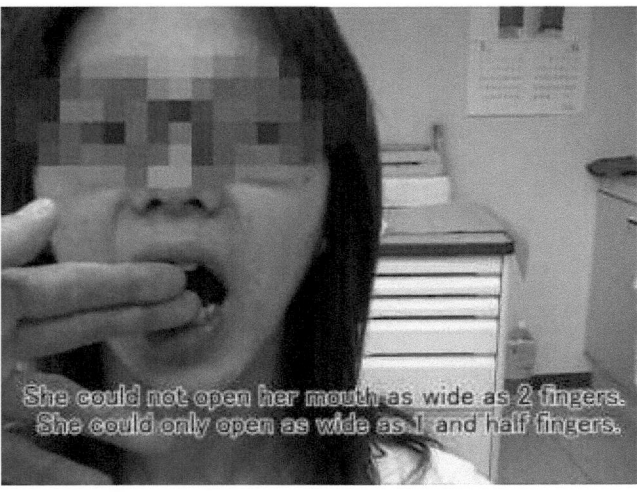

Figure 42: She could open her mouth only as wide as one and half fingers' width before treatment.

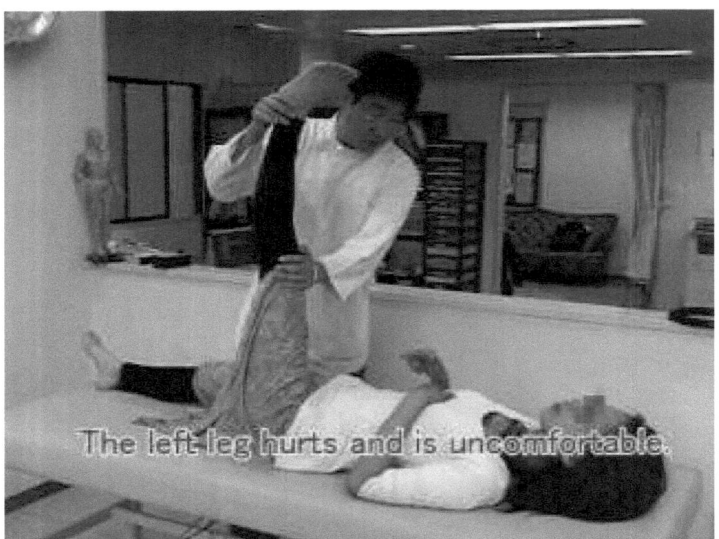

Figure 43: When SLR (Straight Leg Raising) test was done, the patient felt pain and discomfort in her left leg.

When the O-ring test was done, the root cause of her temporomandibular disorder was found to be abnormalities of the joints around the pelvis and the right ankle. This means that the root cause of the temporomandibular disorder was located around her pelvis and ankle. Therefore, before treating the inside of the mouth, these joints should be treated. So, the author used manipulative therapy of AKA (Arthoro-kinematic Approach) on the sacroiliac joint (Figure 44) and the right ankle joint (Figure 45).

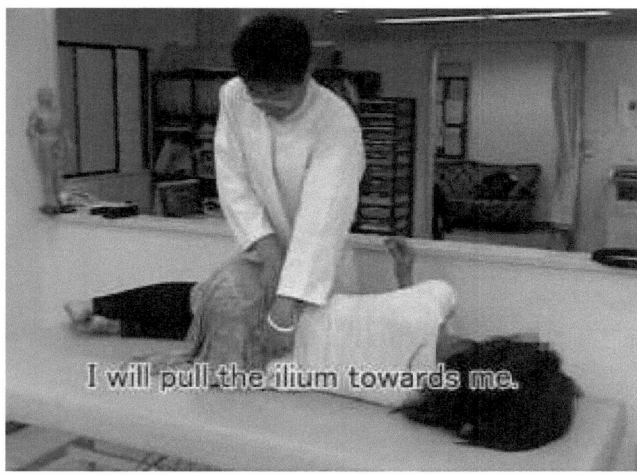

Figure 44: The author used manipulative therapy of AKA on the sacroiliac joint.

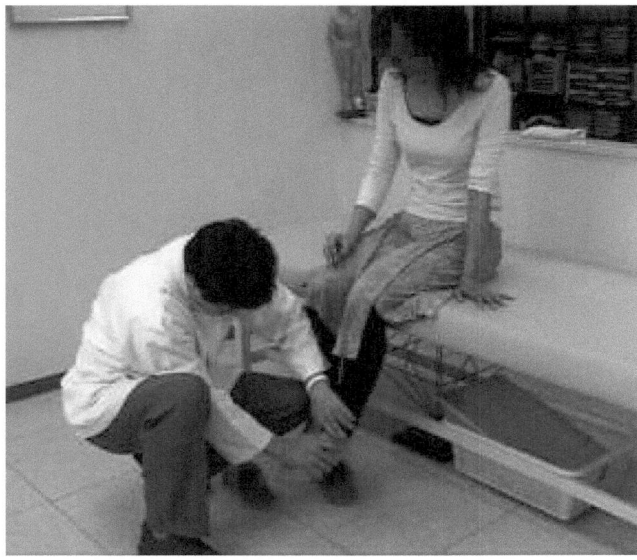

Figure 45: The author used manipulative therapy of AKA on the ankle joint.

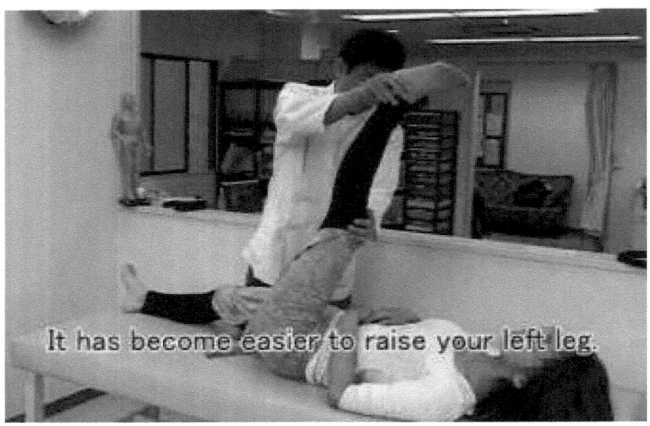

Figure 46: The subject's ability to raise her left leg and open her mouth improved quickly after AKA.

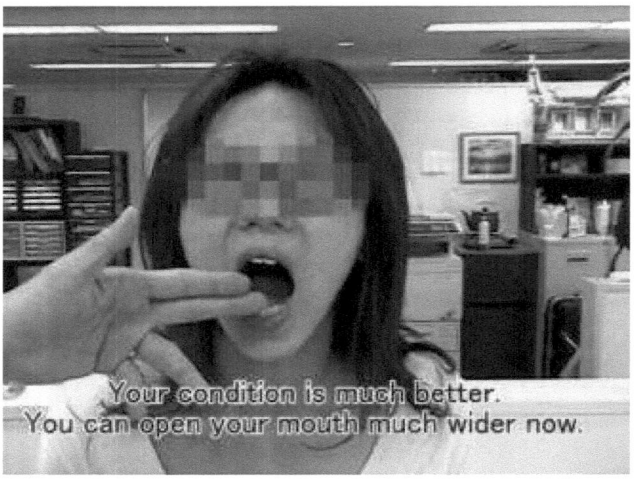

Figure 47: The subject's ability to open her mouth improved and she could open her mouth as wide as three fingers' width quickly after AKA.

After this therapy the subject's ability to raise her left leg and open her mouth improved quickly (Figure 46, 47). Her other TMD symptoms, such as pain in the jaw and clicking also improved. Following the treatment, the subject's dark expression changed completely into a smiling face.

Discussion

If the cause of a chief complaint is a referred symptom, we should treat the original cause first, such as was done in this case. Even if the chief complaint is around the oral area, we should treat outside of the oral area. Thus, if the root cause of the problem is outside of the mouth, the inside of the mouth should not be treated first. Although TMD is defined as a dental ailment, since the cause is often found in other parts of the body, dentists need to learn techniques for performing joint adjustments on other parts of the body, or they need to form cooperative relationships with medical doctors or chiropractic doctors etc. who can perform such treatments. This case is a good example of how dentistry and medicine can be combined.

This concept will be easy to understand if you consider the relationship between shoes and lumbago. If shoes which have uneven wearing at the heels are worn, the length of each leg will be different, and as a result the pelvis may incline, which may result in lumbago. In order to treat this symptom, you need a cobbler, not an orthopedist. The shoes should be improved first because they are the main cause of the problem. If the original cause of TMD is not in the mouth (in this case, the root causes were at the joints around her pelvis and one ankle), we should not try to adjust the teeth or place a mouth piece, because proper biting condition may be destroyed. When we are searching for the root cause or adequate treatment to cure TMD, application of the O-ring test is very convenient.

AKA which was used in this case is a manipulative therapy which mainly improves the condition of articular capsules. I think AKA is very effective but unfortunately this technic is not wide spread. If other technics are effective, they should be used.

Even though Case 9 and the following Case 10 were both temporomandibular disorders, the causes were different. Case 9 was a case in which bite adjustment improved the patient's temporomandibular disorder, as well as shoulder stiffness and headaches. On the other hand, Case 10 was a case in which the patient's temporomandibular disorder was improved by adjusting the joints of the lower body. Since the causes of temporomandibular disorder vary, treatment must also vary. Adequate treatment of temporomandibular disorder cannot be performed if investigation is only done using localized X-ray, MRI, etc. The whole body must be examined.

When treating temporomandibular disorder, it is necessary to attend to the joints throughout the body. Firstly, we can find the part of the body which needs to be treated quickly. Conversely, it tells us which body parts do not need treatment. Furthermore, if the two-point time lag stimulating method, which the author advocates, is used, the body part which should be treated preferentially can be determined. Next, the method for treating the problem area can be chosen.

The O-ring Test can also indicate in which direction a bone should be shifted. Furthermore, it indicates whether further medical treatment is required by allowing us to assess whether there have been any improvements.

In order to watch the actual experiment described in this case, please visit the YouTube movie:

Temporomandibular disorder caused by joint abnormalities in the lower body.

https://www.youtube.com/upload

Case 11

A disorder of the jaw caused backache.

AKA on temporomandibular joints improved the backache, spinal column misalignment, and the inclination of her pelvis.

Subject, Method, and Result

This case involves a 35-year-old woman. She felt discomfort and had dull lower-back pain that had started the day before she came to my office. On the consultation day, her condition got gradually worse and her spinal column became contorted (Figure 48). The orthopedist in charge examined her and she was directed to fix her pelvis with a rubber corset (Figure 49). However, because her waist condition did not improve, she came to my dental clinic later that day. The author treated her temporomandibular joints with AKA (Figure 50). Immediately afterwards, her spinal column misalignment and the inclination of her pelvis improved (Figure 51). Her lumbago also improved. She received an additional simple bite adjustment following her initial treatment. Since then her symptoms have not reccurred.

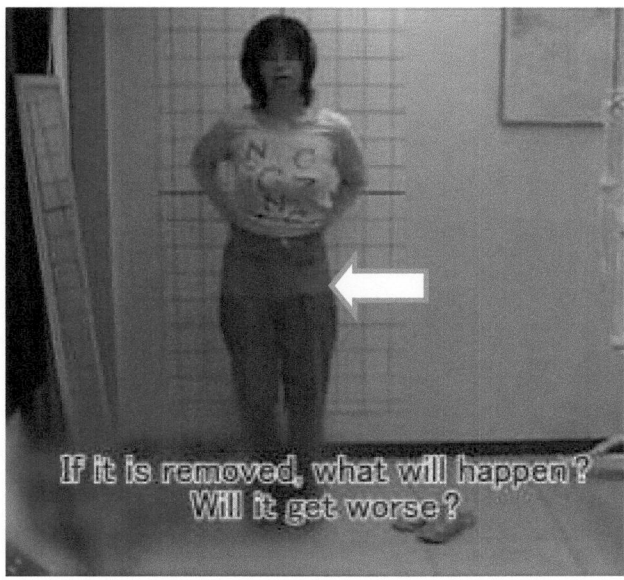

Figure 49: The orthopedist in charge examined her and she was directed to fix her pelvis with a rubber corset (arrow).

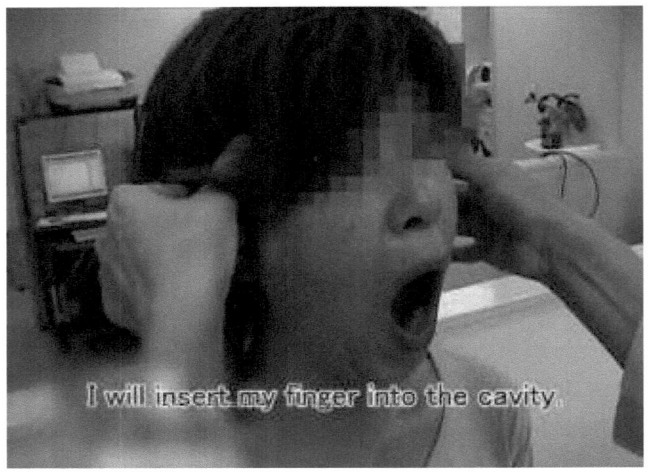

Figure 50: The author treated her temporomandibular joints with AKA.

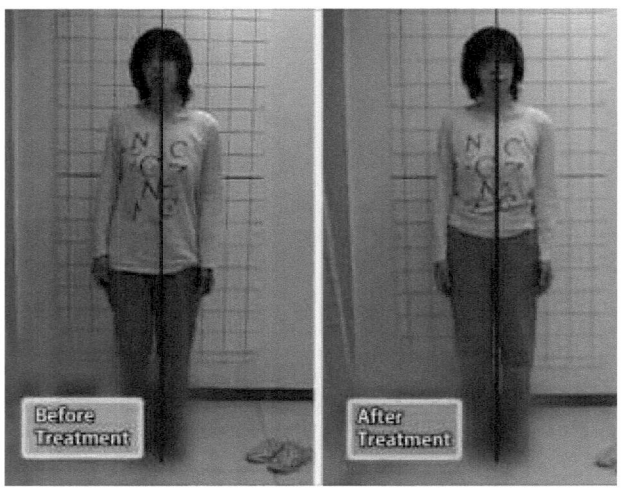

Figure 48   Figure 51

Figure 46: Her spinal column misalignment and the inclination of her pelvis were shown before the treatment.

Figure 51: Her spinal column misalignment and the inclination of her pelvis improved after the treatment.

Discussion

All the joints in the human body are closely related to each other. It seems that the sacroiliac joints and temporomandibular joints have many common features. One pair of sacroiliac joints exists on either side of the sacrum, and the sacrum exists in the center of the body. Conversely, one pair of temporomandibular joints exists on either side of the lower jawbone, and the lower jawbone exists in the center of the body.

Thus, temporomandibular joints and sacroiliac joints have common features which are not found in other joints, so correlations may exist between these joints. Cases 10 and 11 are examples of these correlations and of how such correlations can be used to cure patients. In Case 10, problems with the jaw joints were improve by treating the lower body (i.e. the sacroiliac joint). In Case 11 problems with the pelvis were improved by treating the jaw joint. Jaw joints and the circumference pelvis joints (sacroiliac articulation, hip joint, etc.) have such a close relationship.

In order to watch the actual experiment described in this case, please visit the YouTube movie:

A disorder of the jaw caused a backache

https://www.youtube.com/watch?v=JMyw_hXcXDU&feature=youtu.be

Case 12

Correlation between the jaw joins and the joints of the pelvic area appear clearly,

part 1.

When the patient's leg was raised, her lower jawbone moved right and backward.

Subject and Experiment

The subject was a woman in her 50's. Her biting condition was normal before the experiment (Figure 52). During the SLR (Straight Leg Raising) test, the subject's leg was raised so that the sacroiliac and hip joints moved (Figure 53). Her jaw joints moved simultaneously (Figure 54). When her leg was dropped, her lower jaw returned to its original position. This demonstrates the close relationship between the sacroiliac and the jaw joints.

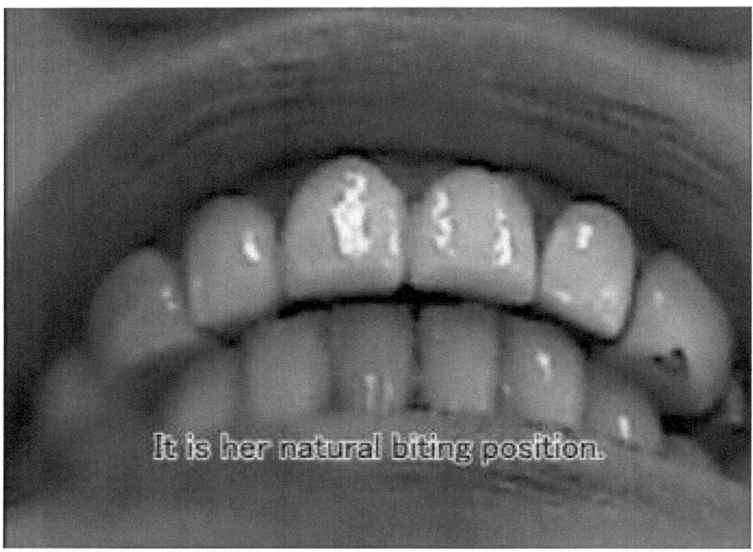

Figure 52: The subject's biting condition was normal before the experiment.

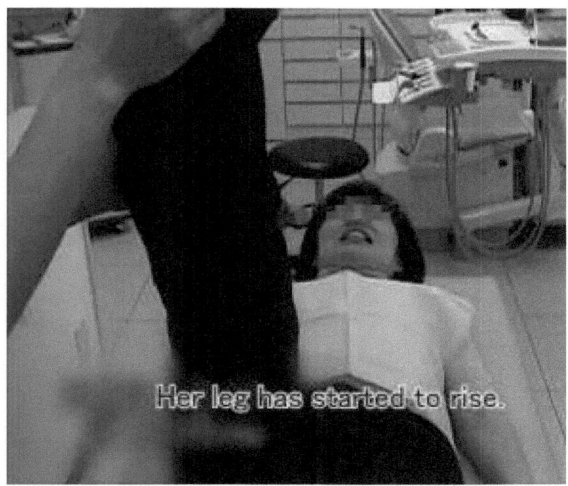

Figure 53: The SLR (Straight Leg Raising) test was performed.

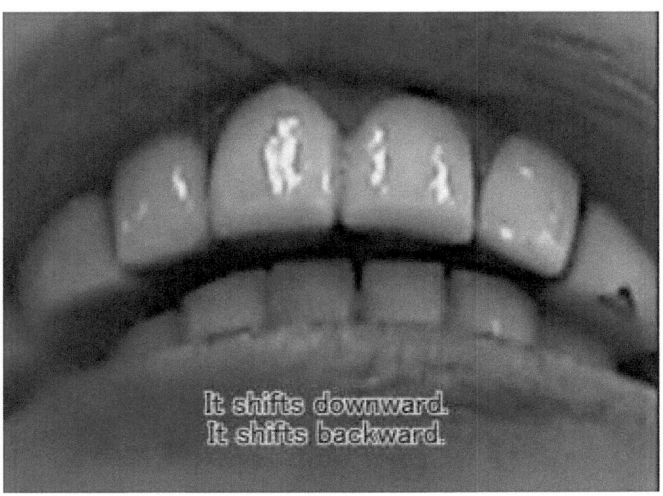

Figure 54: The subject's jaw moved while her leg was being raised.

In order to watch the actual experiment described in this case, please visit the YouTube movie:

Correlation between the jaw joint and the joints of the pelvic area, part 1

https://www.youtube.com/watch?v=lpgDKYvz5_E&feature=youtu.be

Case 13

The correlation between the jaw joints and the joints of the pelvic area appear clearly,

part 2.

When the subject's leg was raised, her lower jawbone shifted to the left.

Subject and Experiment

The subject was a woman in her 20's. When the left leg was raised, the lower jaw shifted to the left (Figure 55). When the leg was dropped, the lower jaw returned to its original position involuntarily (Figure 56).

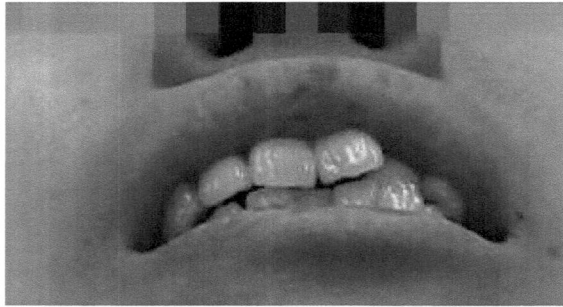

Figure 55: When the left leg was raised, the lower jaw shifted to the left.

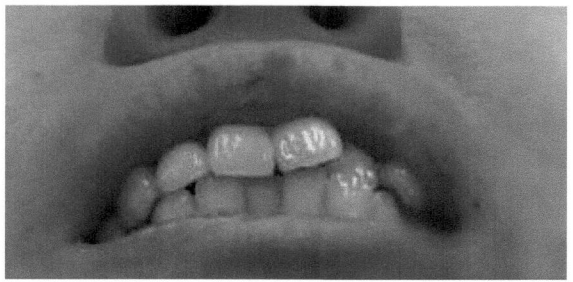

Figure 56: When the leg was dropped, the lower jaw returned to its original position involuntarily.

Discussion

This type of interconnection between the jaw joints and the circumference pelvis joints is rarely as noticeable as it is in these two cases. Therefore, I will describe an experiment that will allow us to understand the correlation between these two joints a little more simply. Please keep about 2mm distance between your upper teeth and lower teeth while sitting on a chair. Then, touch your upper and lower teeth together gently. This is called tapping in dentistry. Try to remember how it feels. Next, cross one leg over the other, then repeat the tapping. I think that you will notice that your jaw has moved slightly. When you cross your leg, the circumference pelvis joint moves. Since the jaw joints are also affected, it seems the two joints are interconnected. Due to this phenomenon, when treating temporomandibular disorder, the circumference pelvis joints should also be diagnosed, and vice versa. Such cases show that the movements of each joint influence other joints. However, in many cases, the medical doctors who treat these interconnected joints have a different specialty, which means these interconnections are missed. The jaw joint is treated by a dentist, while the circumference pelvis joint is treated by orthopedics. In such a situation, it may be difficult to identify the root cause of an ailment. This may lead to the treatment of symptoms, but not the fundamental cause of the problem. Western medicine is focused on local diagnosis and local treatment. Therefore, it is not good at realizing the correlations between different regions of the body. Therefore, I think that holistic medical treatment, which diagnoses and treats the whole body, should be promoted more.

In order to watch the actual experiment described in this case, please visit the YouTube movie:
Correlation between the jaw joint and the joints of the pelvic area, part 2
https://www.youtube.com/watch?v=LJ6zh0MpKRo&feature=youtu.be

Case 14

Soon after extraction of a wisdom tooth, a 60-year-old woman's fingers could reach the floor for the first time.

Subject, Method, and Result

The subject was a 60-year-old woman who used to suffer from lumbago. Her body had been stiff from childhood. When she bent from the waist, she was unable to bring her fingers within 10 cm of the floor (Figure 57).

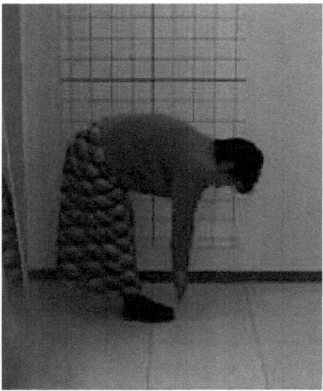

Figure 57: When she bent from the waist, she was unable to bring her fingers within 10 cm of the floor

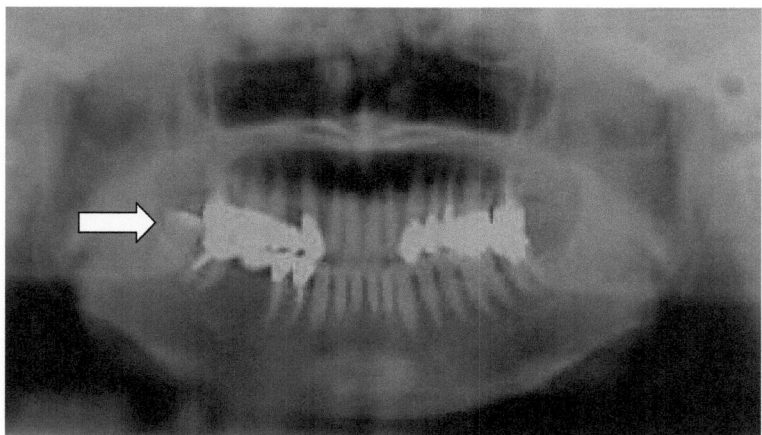

Figure 58: Using the O-ring test, it became clear that movement of the jaw was being interrupted owing to her lower right wisdom tooth, which had grown in (arrow).

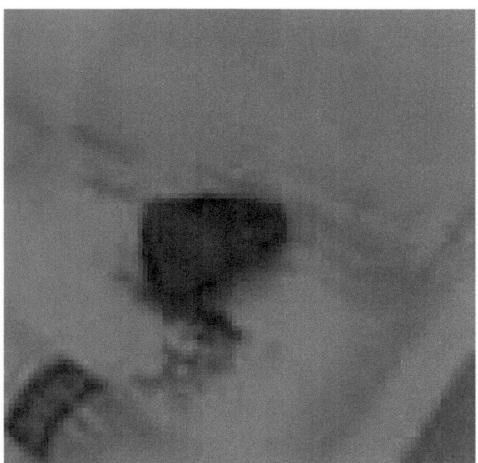

Figure 59: Extracted right lower wisdom tooth.

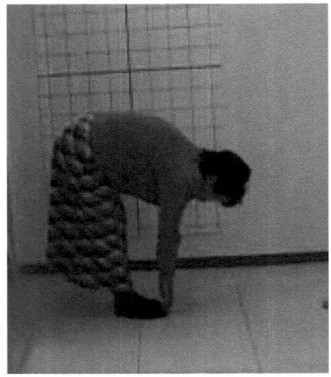

Figure 60: She was able to touch the floor with her fingers while bending at the waist after the wisdom tooth removal.

Using the O-ring test, it became clear that movement of the jaw was being interrupted owing to her lower right wisdom tooth (Figure 58), which had grown in. The wisdom tooth was pulled out (Figure 59). Subsequently, she was able to touch the floor with her fingers while bending at the waist. "I have reached the floor for the first time in my life at the age of 60", she said. Evidently, her lumbago had improved.

Discussion

Although the body seems to become stiff with age, it may usually be rejuvenated in an instant after dental care like the treatment described above. If a tooth does not have an opposing tooth, it may grow out more than usual. This will result in a gap between it, and the next tooth. When the height of teeth is different, it may affect jaw movement. It becomes hard to open the mouth or to move the jaw. This may cause lumbago. The above mentioned condition is often seen with wisdom teeth. The wisdom tooth that I extracted from the subject did not have an opposing tooth. Therefore, her wisdom tooth overgrew, so that it extended past the teeth next to it. This seemed to negatively affect her ability to bite properly.

In order to watch the actual experiment described in this case, please visit the YouTube movie:

A 60-year-old woman's fingers could reach the floor for the first time.

https://www.youtube.com/watch?v=dga3lZdfh64&feature=youtu.be

Case 15

Backache improved after extraction of a wisdom tooth

Subject, Method, and Result

The subject was a 20-year-old woman who suffer from backaches if she stood for a long period of time. When the SLR test was done, the left leg could only be raised to 80 degrees, and when the knee was adducted, there was pain in her hip joint (Figure 61). When investigated by the O-ring test, it turned out that her upper right wisdom tooth (Figure 62) stimulated the membrane inside her cheek (buccal mucous membrane), and that this stimulation was connected with her lumbago. Therefore, her upper right wisdom tooth was pulled out (Figure 63). When the SLR test was done again, the pain in her hip joint had disappeared and the joint's mobility had increased as well. Her circumference pelvis joints (sacroiliac articulation and hip joint) had become more flexible (Figure 64). In addition, she happily reported that her shoulders felt better and that the condition of her back had become better, too. However, compared to the last case, it took more time for the joint mobility to improve.

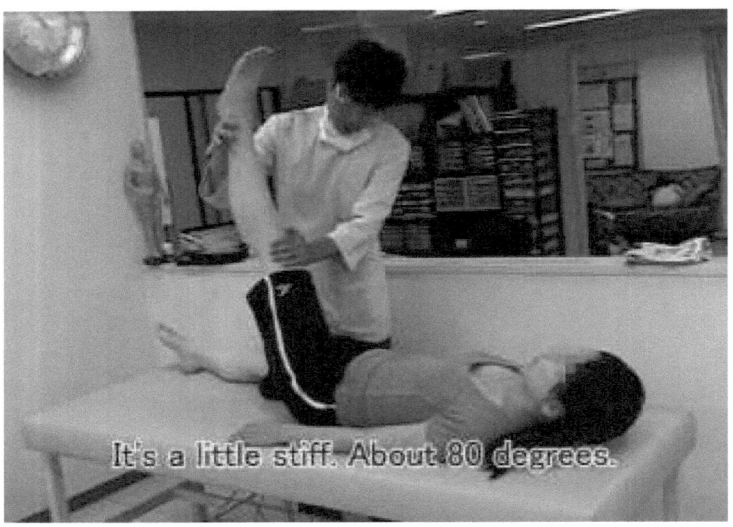

Figure 61: When the SLR test was done, the left leg could only be raised to 80 degrees.

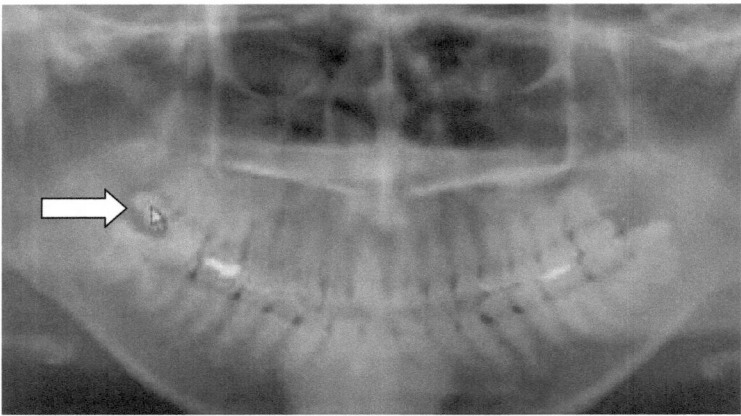

Figure 62: When investigated by the O-ring test, it turned out that her upper right wisdom tooth (arrow) stimulated the membrane inside her cheek.

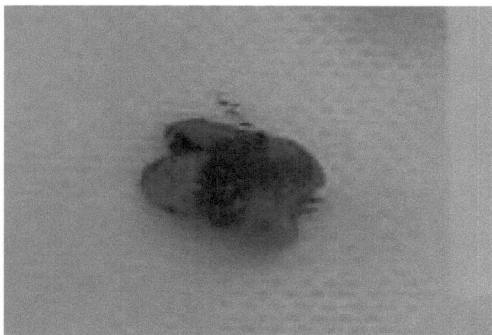

Figure 63: The removed upper right wisdom tooth.

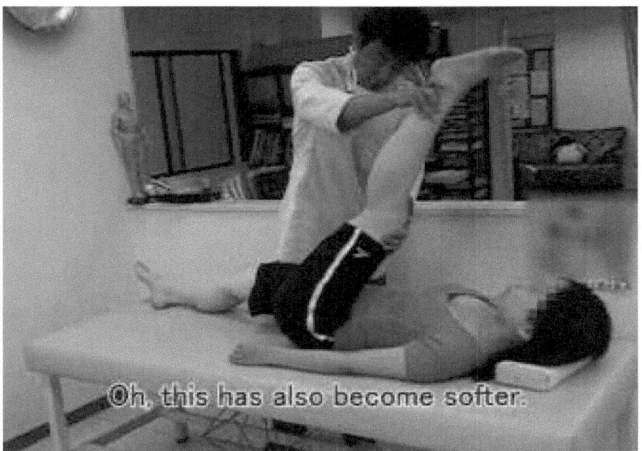

Figure 64: When the SLR test was done, the left leg could now be raised to 120 degrees.

Discussion

In Cases 14 and 15, I pulled out wisdom teeth which did not have opposing teeth. This can be seen clearly on the X-rays in the movie. Even though these teeth did not make contact with other teeth during biting, they still caused systemic symptoms. This may indicate that bite stimulation is not the only cause of systemic symptoms. It may also be related to position or membrane stimulation, etc. In order to confirm the root cause of such symptoms, I use the O-ring test. Some patients will respond immediately after treatment, others need some minutes to respond, other may take hours or days, while others do not respond at all. Moreover, there are those who are aware of changes in their body condition immediately, while others who are not as sensitive to such changes. It is not clear why reactions after treatment are different from person to person. I think that people react differently to such treatment due to variations in sensitivity to systemic changes i.e. sensitivity to pain or stiffness. However, more research needs to be done. In the future, I hope to be able to clarify the reasons for such variation in sensitivity and ultimately to be able to modify people's sensitivity. If a person is not sensitive enough, they will wait too long for treatment, but if they are over-sensitive, it is difficult to live a normal life. By creating the ideal level of sensitivity in each person, I hope to be able to more easily assess and treat the root causes of a wide variety of ailments (i.e. atopic dermatitis, allergies, chemical sensitivity, etc.)

Treatment utilizing electromagnetic waves emitted from substances. Each substance emits particular electromagnetic waves. These waves can have an influence on the body. This concept is not widely accepted by modern science, but it can be demonstrated by the O-ring test. If a substance which emits particular electromagnetic waves is brought close to the body, it is possible to treat ailments without touching the body or administering medicine. Qi-gong, or the laying of hands on the sick, may be an example of how the electromagnetic waves emitted by the human body can be used to treat ailments. Systemic symptoms are induced by wisdom teeth. It is said that modern human beings have a small jaw because of changing habits. It is common for there to not be enough space for wisdom teeth sprouting, so wisdom teeth often come in unusually. As a result, wisdom teeth stimulate the membrane of the cheek unusually. Such unusual stimulation may induce systemic symptoms. Let's examine such a case.

In order to watch the actual experiment described in this case, please visit the YouTube movie:

Backache improvement after extraction of a wisdom tooth
https://www.youtube.com/watch?v=EekTPdMufkc&feature=youtu.be

Case 16

The electromagnetic waves emitted by a dental crown influence the whole body.

A crown set under a patient's foot improved lumbago.

Subject, Method, and Result

The subject was a 50-year-old woman who was worried about intense lumbago. Whatever she tried, she was not able to find a successful treatment until she visited my dental clinic after being referred by a medical doctor. Although she could walk by herself, she was hardly able to bend her body forwards or backwards (Figure 65, 66).Utilizing the O-ring test, I was able to determine that her biting situation was almost normal, but that the metal used in the crown that covered her upper right first molar was having a negative influence on her body. Subsequently, the crown was removed and a crown made of gold and platinum alloy was manufactured. Before the crown was set in her mouth, it was placed under her foot. After that, her lumbago improved and she was able to bend forward and backward easily. However, when the crown was covered with aluminum foil to block the electromagnetic waves, her lumbago returned and she could hardly bend. When this crown was set in her mouth, her lumbago almost completely disappeared. The lumbago, which had been continuously worrying her for a long time, was cured utilizing only this common dental treatment.

Discussion

This is a very important case, because it shows how particular electromagnetic waves affect the body. I first noticed the influence of electromagnetic waves when I examined a patient with knee pain several years ago. I thought the cause of the patient's knee pain was her denture. I removed the patient's denture and scraped the sharp portion.

When I had almost finished reshaping the denture, the patient, who had been continually complaining of pain, said that the pain had disappeared. I thought it was unbelievable because her denture was not yet placed in her mouth yet. When I moved the denture away from her, she said that her knee pain returned. When the denture was brought close to the body again, the pain disappeared once more. This incident led me to notice how different substances emit unique electromagnetic waves. I have repeated this process with many substances. The results are usually similar; I encourage you to try it as well. For example, please compare how far forward you can bend when you place a banana underfoot to how far forward you can bend with a pineapple underfoot.

Please repeat this experiment using other substances. I think that many people will experience variations in how far forward they can bend. This demonstrates how the body can be influenced by external substances. This phenomenon can be shown using the O-ring test. Grip strength changes when substances are brought close to the body.

I think it better for overall health, if the amount of flexibility is increased. Please stir your coffee or tea clockwise or counter-clockwise. Please place the clockwise rotating liquid underfoot or the counter-clockwise rotating liquid underfoot. Then, compare how far you can bend. I think that many people's ability to bend forward will vary depending on the direction of rotation. Moreover, many people will notice that the taste is different as well. Direction of rotation does not alter the liquid's matter. However, the reaction of a living body differs. The reasons why this phenomenon happens cannot be explained scientifically. Modern science is in a developing state, which cannot even explain such a simple natural phenomenon. So, it is not right to say that since there is scientific evidence, something is true but that since there is no scientific evidence, something is false.

In order to watch the actual experiment described in this case, please visit the YouTube movie:

Lumbago improves by simply placing a crown near foot

https://www.youtube.com/watch?v=FoTSWuVw24s

Case 17

A patient's lumbago improved when Chinese medicine was brought close to her body.

Subject, Method, and Result

The subject was a woman in her 40's who was troubled by lumbago. In the hospital, her lumbago was diagnosed as a herniated disc. When an MRI was done, it turned out that an intervertebral disc had come out. The subject could not walk because of the intense pain, so I went to her house to perform the treatment. She was not able to stand up straight because of her lumbago. Using the O-ring test, I selected which Chinese medicine (Chinese herbal extract preparation) would work for the subject's lumbago, and placed it at the base of her neck. Subsequently, the pain in her back improved and she could stand up straight without any other treatment. She said that she felt like the medicine was pulling her, so that her back straightened without any conscious effort.

As soon as the medicine was removed, her back became painful again and she was not able to keep her posture upright. I recommended that the subject place the Chinese medicine on her mattress, then cover it with a sheet so that she could sleep close the medicine. She said that her lumbago became better when she was sleeping.

Discussion

Modern Western medical science believes that medicine cannot be effective unless it is absorbed into the body. It uses tests such as the Cohort examination and blind studies to determine the effectiveness of medicines. However, there may be a problem with these tests. They assume that medicines or placebos that are close to the body, but not administered, have no influence. This is wrong. As was discussed in Case 17, medicine can have an influence on the body without being absorbed by the body. This is caused by the electromagnetic waves emitted by the medicines. I think that it is dangerous to accept the experimental data that have been obtained from modern scientific methods because the phenomenon discussed above may be influencing results. Furthermore, in modern medicine, it is believed that the same substance will produce the same effect on the body consistently. However, as I showed above, the same substance (i.e. coffee or tea) can have a different effect on the body depending on which way it is rotating. The taste may change, and body flexibility may change, simply by bringing the liquid close to the body. Therefore, when taking medicine, the effect of a medicine may differ depending on whether the water used to swallow the medicine is rotating clockwise or counter-clockwise. Current Western medicine does not consider such a concept at all. Therefore, just as in Case 17, medicine may be effective when it is placed into bedding, or kept in a pocket. These alternative methods of drug administration may be just as effective and may also prevent side-effects. For example, there are patients who cannot continue to receive anti-cancer drugs because the side effects are too strong. However, if the drug is near the cancer, the patient may receive the benefits of the drug without side-effects. There is a story that when Christ placed his hand on an ailment, it improved. It might have been the result of the particular electromagnetic waves emitted by Christ's hand.

In order to watch the actual experiment described in this case, please visit the YouTube movie:
Lumbago was improved by the indirect effect of medicine
https://www.youtube.com/watch?v=TmiAatOdHhU

Case 18

Neck pain and stiffness are improved by bringing an antibiotic close to the body.

Subject, Method, and Result

The subject was a woman in her 50's who had complained of her head being sore and difficult to turn. Although she could turn her head to the right fairly well, it was difficult to turn it to the left because of pain and stiffness. Since a suppurative lesion of the upper right bicuspid was suspected to be the cause, as determined by the O-ring test, an antibiotic was placed on the outer surface of her right cheek. As a result, it became easier to turn her head to the left. When the medicine was removed from her cheek, the pain and stiffness returned and it was once more difficult for her to turn her head to the left.

Discussion

This phenomenon is likely due to electromagnetic waves. The pain and stiffness in the patient's neck, which were caused by pathogenic bacteria, were neutralized by the electromagnetic waves emitted by the antibiotic when it was brought close to the infected area.

In order to watch the actual experiment described in this case, please visit the YouTube movie:
Neck pain and stiffness are improved by bringing an antibiotic close to the body.
https://www.youtube.com/watch?v=IsOnh4vpOBM

Case 19

Frozen shoulder, which normally takes a long time to cure, is improved after a single dental treatment

Subject, Method, and Result

The subject was a woman in her 50's who had a shoulder that suddenly became sore three days before coming to my clinic. The base of her left shoulder was painful and she could not raise her left arm more than 10 cm from her side (Figure 65). After the O-ring test, it turned out that there was a problem with her upper denture, so the denture was adjusted. She said that the treatment only caused a small improvement during the first day after treatment. However, it gradually became easier to raise her arm from the evening of the day after treatment. When she visited my clinic two weeks later, her shoulder pain was completely gone and she had full use of her left arm (Figure 66).

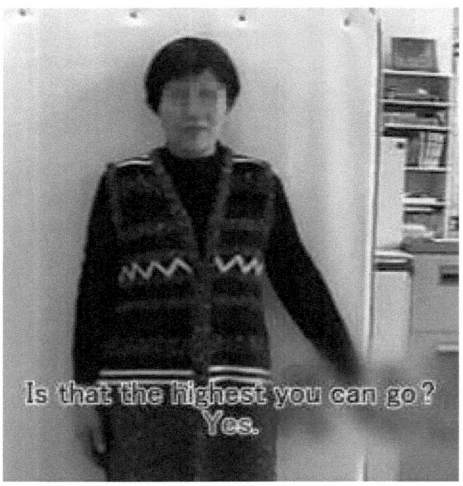

Figure 65: The base of her left shoulder was painful and she could not raise her left arm more than 10 cm from her side

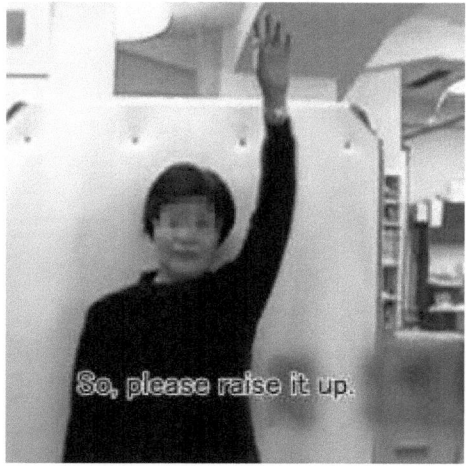

Figure 66: Her shoulder pain was completely gone and she had full use of her left arm two weeks after treatment.

In this case, there was little change in the patient's condition immediately after dental treatment. The full effect of the treatment was felt from the second day. However, in some cases, notable improvement may be felt immediately after dental treatment. This ailment is common, but not easily cured. Frozen shoulder, knee pain, hip joint pain, lumbago, etc. are common conditions which many people have experienced at least once. However, orthopedic treatments may be ineffective and manual therapeutics and massage are just temporary solutions. In addition, recovery can take from several months to several years. Moreover, the condition may reoccur after the initial recovery. Dental care may succeed in treating these conditions.

In order to watch the actual experiment described in this case, please visit the YouTube movie:

Frozen shoulder is improved after a single dental treatment

https://www.youtube.com/watch?v=1lytPdwyTZM&feature=youtu.be

Case 20

Common knee pain can be improved by dental treatment in several seconds.

Subject, Method, and Result

The subject was a woman in her 50's who had pain in her right knee for two weeks before she came for treatment. She was not able to bend down or stand up well. As she bent down, she began to feel pain when her thigh and shin were at 90 degrees. Moreover, it was so painful that she could not stand up without supporting herself with her hands. When a little occlusal surface of the lower right first premolar was scraped, the pain in her knees disappeared, and it became easier for her to bend down and stand up.

Discussion

Arthritic pain in the knees is common in middle-aged people. In many cases, doctors say there is not much they can do. It is just a result of getting older. Patients are told to reduce their weight or to do muscle strengthening exercises. Operations may be recommended when the condition is severe. ADL (activities of daily living) can fall gradually due to pain in the knees, and some patients may become bedridden. Biting condition may be the root cause of such knee pain. Therefore, a single tooth adjustment may lead to a full recovery in cases such as the one discussed above (Case 20).

In order to watch the actual experiment described in this case, please visit the YouTube movie:
Knee pain is reduced after a single treatment which only took several seconds
https://www.youtube.com/watch?v=QhVMvFrqa2c

Case 21

Treatment of degenerative hip disease by irradiating the palate with a soft laser

Subject, Method, and Result

The subject was a woman in her 60's who had difficulty walking due to hip joint pain. It was diagnosed as degenerative hip disease and an operation was recommended. When the SLR test was done, her left leg rose to 60 degrees but her right leg could not be raised at all. She could not bend her left leg outward at all, either. When the cause was investigated by the O-ring test, it turned out that her skull was likely to have morbid modification. So, I irradiated her palate with a soft laser often used for the dental treatment of stomatitis or dentin hypersensitivity. After this treatment, her hip joints became flexible. In the SLR test, both of her legs raised to 90 degrees. As for outer bending, her knee could bend to touch the bed's surface. Since completing this treatment, she has felt no pain while walking or exercising.

Discussion

The relationship between the cranium and sacrum is well known in chiropractic medicine. The stress build up in her palate was affecting her hip joint. As a result of improving her cranial distortion with the soft laser, it seems that the condition of the hip joint also improved. Soft lasers are often used to treat dental hypersensitivity or stomatitis. There is no pain during irradiation and it is also safe for the body.

In order to watch the actual experiment described in this case, please visit the YouTube movie:
Treatment of degenerative hip disease by irradiating the palate with a soft laser
https://www.youtube.com/watch?v=MA8NrccufqA

Case 22

Hip joint flexibility and balance improved after orthodontic treatment which was guided by the O-ring test

Subject, Method, and Result

The subject was a ten-year-old girl who wanted to be a ballerina. She was not able to raise her left leg as high above her head as her right leg, due to reduced flexibility in her left hip joint (Figure 67, 68). Since the abnormal position of the lower right front teeth was judged to be the root cause of the problem (Figure 69), using the O-ring test, an orthodontic appliance was attached right away. Just after attaching the appliance, although the teeth had not yet moved, the motion of her left hip joint became better, and she was able to raise her left leg as high as her right. After additional dental treatment (Figure 70), she was able to touch the side of her head with both her left and right legs (Figure 71, 72). Her sense of balance also improved, so she was able to pause with one of her legs in the air, which she had not been able to do well before. This orthodontic treatment was not only performed for aesthetic reasons (Figure 73), but was done to enhance the patient's ability to do ballet. However, as a result of the treatment, the alignment of her teeth also improved. The result of this case illustrates how the O-ring test can be used with orthodontic treatment to improve overall health as well as oral health.

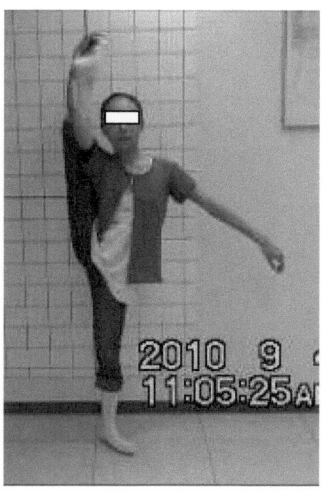

Figure 67: The subject was able to raise her right leg higher than her left leg.

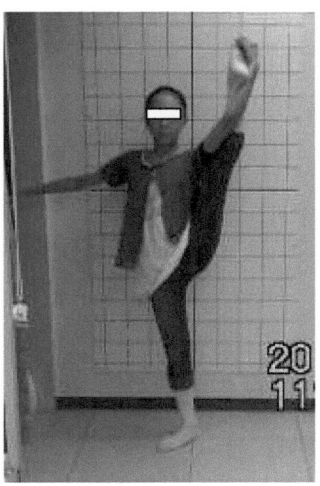

Figure 68: The subject was not able to raise her left leg as high above her head as her right leg, due to reduced flexibility in her left hip joint.

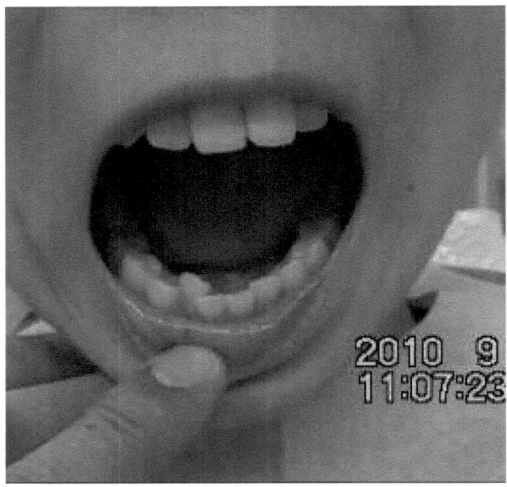

Figure 69: The abnormal position of the lower right front teeth was judged to be the root cause of the problem.

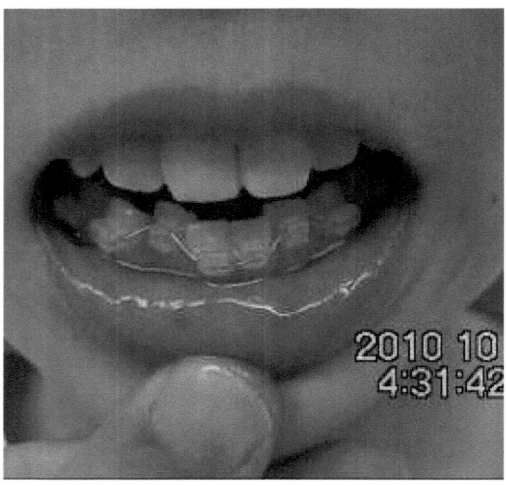

Figure 70: An orthodontic appliance was attached.

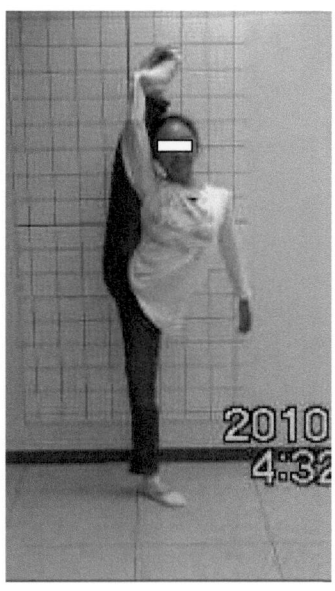

Figure 71: The subject was able to touch the side of her head with her right leg.

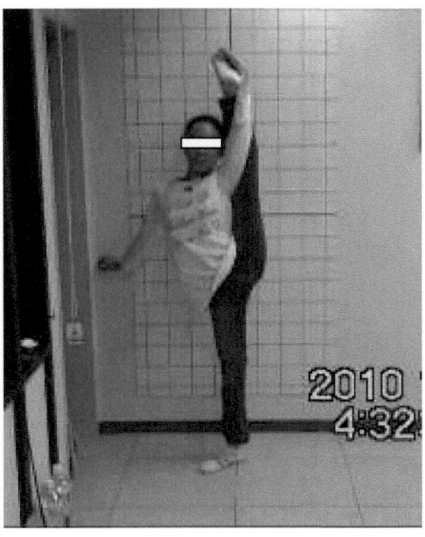

Figure 72: The subject was able to touch the side of her head with both legs.

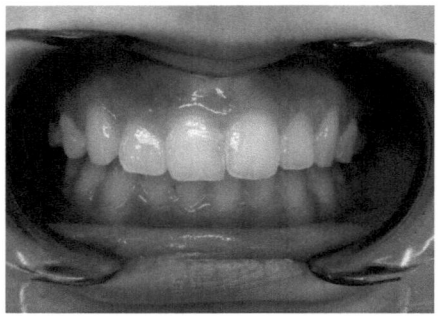

Figure 73: The subject's lower front teeth were properly aligned about three years after initial orthodontic treatment. She has continued to experience the positive results of this treatment

Discussion

I found that the cause of the patient's hip joint stiffness was the misalignment of her lower front teeth. I advocate using the two-point time lag stimulating method to uncover such relationships, since it allows us to judge the cause and effect between two related points in the body. However, there are several O-ring test methods, so more research needs to be done to find the best method. Many people are troubled by stiffness. Owing to stiffness, some people develop lumbago and shoulder problems. Many of these people stretch every day to relieve their stiffness. These people should be careful, because their stiffness may be a signal from the body telling them to avoid dangerous movements. In fact, some patients come to my clinic with damage from over-stretching.

As the DVD shows, it is possible for body flexibility to improve after appropriate dental treatment. In such cases, stretching is not necessary to improve flexibility. This phenomenon results from a change in the signals that the body sends after dental treatment. After the oral disorder is treated, the body stops sending signals not to bend, which allows the patient to move more freely. I predict that further research will lead to the discovery of a mechanism that allows oral disorders to instruct the brain to restrict body movement, since treatment of oral disorders has been shown to improve joint flexibility.

In order to watch the actual experiment described in this case, please visit the YouTube movie:
Orthodontic treatment to improve hip joint mobility and balance
https://www.youtube.com/watch?v=MjkmVjXxTEo

Case 23

A mouthpiece is used not only to protect the body but also to increase sports performance

Experiment

The subject was a man in his 20's and an American football player. Two temporary mouthpieces, which resulted in different biting positions, were made for this case. One resulted in a 3mm gap between the upper and lower incisors when it was worn. The other resulted in a 3mm gap between the incisors and shifted the jaw horizontally so that the O-ring was closed. I inserted each mouthpiece and then arm wrestled him. The difference in his strength when wearing one of the two mouthpieces was clear. I was able to defeat the subject when he was wearing the first mouthpiece, which did not shift his bite horizontally (Figure 74), because he could not generate enough power. However, when he was wearing the second mouthpiece, which was made using the results of the O-ring test, he showed a remarkable increase in power and easily defeated me (Figure 75).

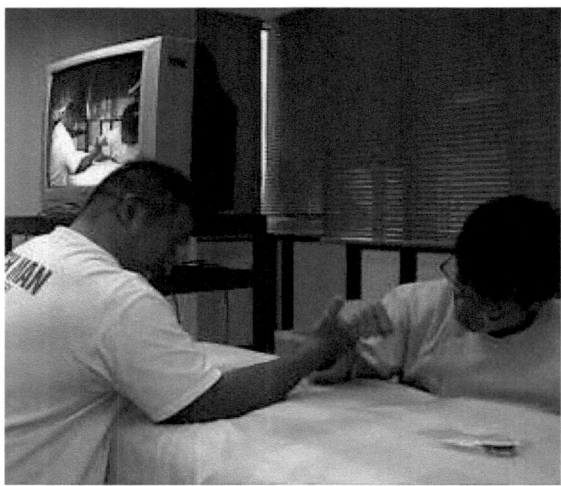

Figure 74: The author (on the right) was able to defeat the subject (on the left) when he was wearing the first mouthpiece, which did not shift his bite horizontally.

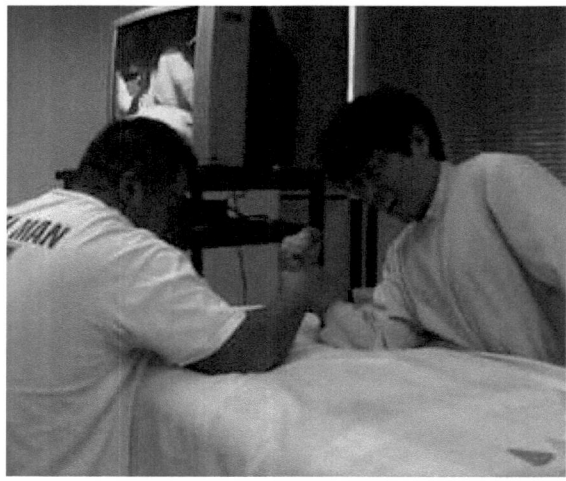

Figure 75: When the subject was wearing the second mouthpiece, which shifted his bite horizontally, he showed a remarkable increase in strength and easily defeated the author.

Discussion

Currently, mouthpieces are used by boxers and other athletes mainly as a way to reduce injuries. However, this case demonstrates that mouthpieces also influence sport performance. Therefore, mouthpieces must be carefully made so as not to reduce sport performance, but to maximize it. In order to do this, it is important to determine the ideal biting position. The O-ring test should be used to do this. Biting treatment should be used in the world of sports. Biting treatment is useful, not only to cure physical ailments, but also to improve overall sports performance. I am one of the researchers studying sports dentistry. I have repeatedly seen examples of how an athlete's personal best can be extended by improving his/her biting condition. I have frequently noted improved power, flexibility and balance following adjustment of a patient's biting condition. Such treatment could be used to improve the performance of international athletes, so sports dentistry should be promoted at the state level.

In order to watch the actual experiment described in this case, please visit the YouTube movie:
A mouthpiece is used not only to protect the body but also to increase sports performance
https://www.youtube.com/watch?v=KroKjl5ODnc

Overall Conclusion

After reading this book, how do you feel about the relationship between dentistry and the whole body? I think you can see how deeply dentistry effects the whole body. As I have pointed out, there are many ailments which Western medicine cannot currently cure. This is because Western medicine only analyzes the parts of the body where the symptoms appear. I am sure that you can understand that if abnormalities in the oral area are the root cause of the illness, medical doctors may not be able to determine such root causes without the cooperation of dentists. Despite such evidence, moves to unite medicine and dentistry are seldom made. Although cooperation between medicine and dentistry is positively advocated by the dentistry side, presently, there are few signs that the medical side is responding. I have two hopes for the future: first, I hope that more and more dentists will use my treatment methods to improve the overall health of their patients, and second, I hope that dentistry and medicine will increase their cooperation, with the ultimate goal of unifying into a single field.

The application of the 2 points time lag stimulation method

I think the Bi-Digital O-Ring Test (Herein, BDORT) is necessary to medical progress, but the permeation seems slow. The reason for this is complicated, but a fundamental principle underlying BDORT is that 'When the body experiences a stimulus in an affected area, the grip is weakened' or 'When something harmful approaches the body the grip weakens'. The affected areas are divided into the symptom and the cause, and it is possible to give priority to treatment of the cause more effectively than the symptom. I believe it's beneficial, so I'd like to introduce.

Method

Affected areas are looked for using BDORT and the order of priority of treatment for these affected areas is decided. For example, when a patient exhibits two affected areas (point A and point B), treatment of the causal point (point A) will remove the need for treatment of the symptom (point B).

When there are two affected areas in the body, each point reveals its abnormalities through the O-ring test (the O-ring opens). Therefore, when stimulating point A, subject's O-ring would open (Herein ORT-), and the opposite is true of point B.

Next, when stimulating point B just after stimulating point A, if ORT- and when stimulating point A just after point B, if the subject's O-ring closes (Herein, ORT+) it is judged that point A holds influence over point B. Therefore, it is judged that point A would be the dominant point for treatment.

Next, when stimulating point B just after stimulating point A, if ORT+ and when stimulating point A just after point B, if ORT+ it is judged that there is no relationship of cause and effect between point A and B. Therefore, it is judged that both points should be treated individually.

Next, when stimulating point B just after stimulating point A, if ORT-and when stimulating point A just after point B, if ORT-it is judged that both points influence each other. In such a case, the author treated the point which produces the weakest grip.

Discussion

When put into practice, this law reveals the dominant area of treatment. The patient's temporal physical load is small, and recurrence will be unlikely. There are also many unclear issues, but I think this phenomenon reflects the flow of Qi, like in Oriental medicine. Now I am attempting to simplify this method.

Therefore, although this method is not accepted now, it would be a useful tool with which to find diagnosis. In the future, this method may help determine the cause and effect of various cancers or autoimmune immunity diseases.

Conclusion

Before recognizing this method as a viable tool, more trials are needed, but I believe it's a remarkable way to trace a chain of cause and effect.

In order to watch the actual experiment described in this case, please visit the YouTube movie:

The two point time lag stimulation method by means of Bi Digital O Ring Test

https://www.youtube.com/watch?v=3DG9hYGEZpc

need for treatment of the symptom (point B).

When there are two affected areas in the body, each point reveals its abnormalities through the O-ling test (the O-ring opens). Therefore, when stimulating point A, the subject's O-ring would open (Herein ORT-

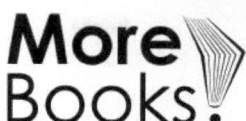
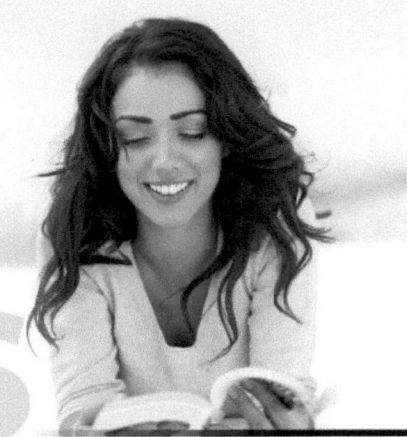

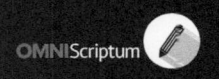

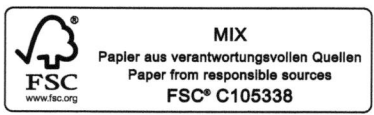